Extraordinary Measures

EXTRAORDINARY MEASURES

Disability in Music

Joseph N. Straus

OXFORD
UNIVERSITY PRESS

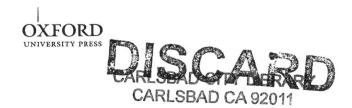

OXFORD
UNIVERSITY PRESS

Oxford University Press, Inc., publishes works that further
Oxford University's objective of excellence
in research, scholarship, and education.

Oxford   New York
Auckland   Cape Town   Dar es Salaam   Hong Kong   Karachi
Kuala Lumpur   Madrid   Melbourne   Mexico City   Nairobi
New Delhi   Shanghai   Taipei   Toronto

With offices in
Argentina   Austria   Brazil   Chile   Czech Republic   France   Greece
Guatemala   Hungary   Italy   Japan   Poland   Portugal   Singapore
South Korea   Switzerland   Thailand   Turkey   Ukraine   Vietnam

Copyright © 2011 Joseph N. Straus

Published by Oxford University Press, Inc.
198 Madison Avenue, New York, New York 10016

www.oup.com

Oxford is a registered trademark of Oxford University Press

Library of Congress Cataloging-in-Publication Data
Straus, Joseph Nathan.
Extraordinary measures : disability in music / Joseph N. Straus.
p.   cm.
Includes bibliographical references and index.
ISBN 978-0-19-976645-1 (hardback)   ISBN 978-0-19-976646-8 (pbk.)
1. Music—Philosophy and aesthetics.   2. Composers with disabilities.
3. Musicians with disabilities.   4. Music—Psychological aspects.
5. Musical analysis.   I. Title.
ML3800.S885 2011
780.87—dc22
2010015826

1 3 5 7 9 8 6 4 2
Printed in the United States of America

For Sally, Adam, and especially Mike

TABLE OF CONTENTS

ACKNOWLEDGMENTS

In the spring of 2002, I found myself riding an Amtrak train back home from Penn State, where I had given a lecture on some musical topic. I fell into conversation with the person sitting next to me—she turned out to be a fellow academic, a professor of literature at Penn State, named Susan Squier. When our conversation died down, I took out a book to read, a book about autism. The eldest of my two sons, Michael, is autistic (he was then ten years old) and like so many concerned parents, I was doing my best to learn about a topic that was, and still is, shrouded in mystery and misinformation. Susan saw what I was reading, and asked if I was interested in "Disability Studies." I replied, "What's that?" At that moment, when Susan started to answer my question, my education about disability as a theoretical, social, and cultural phenomenon began.

At Susan's suggestion, I started to read the foundational texts in Disability Studies, by Paul Longmore, Simi Linton, Lennard Davis, Rosemarie Garland-Thomson, and others, and as my excitement at this new way of thinking about disability mounted, I began to wonder about its implications for music. Other than some pioneering work by Alex Lubet, there was no disability-related scholarship on music to turn to, and so to begin to sort through the issues, I organized a panel discussion at a meeting of the American Musicological Society in Seattle in 2004. This marked the entrance of Disability Studies onto the main stage of North American musicology, and the participants on that panel (Maria Cizmic, Brian Hyer, Marianne Kielian-Gilbert, Neil Lerner, Jay Rahn, and Amy Vidali) have formed the nucleus of a small but growing community that has sustained me ever since. Several of the participants later contributed to a collection of essays I coedited with Neil Lerner (*Sounding Off: Theorizing Disability in Music*, Routledge 2006), the first such collection in this area.

Since then, we have seen, perhaps not a torrent, but a steady stream of publications on the cultural construction of disability in music. I wrote an article in the *Journal of the American Musicological Society* ("Normalizing the Abnormal: Disability in Music and Music Theory," Straus 2006a) that forms the basis of chapters 2, 3, and 6 of this book. I am grateful to the friends and colleagues who read that article when it was in draft and made valuable suggestions (Charles Burkhart, James Gleick, Sally Goldfarb,

Ellie Hisama, Brian Hyer, Richard Kramer, Shaugn O'Donnell, and Starry Schor) and to the editors of that journal for permitting me to reprint parts of it here. My essay in *Sounding Off* ("Inversional Balance and the 'Normal' Body in the Music of Arnold Schoenberg and Anton Webern," Straus 2006b) forms the basis of chapter 4, and an article in the *Journal of Musicology* ("Disability and Late Style in Music," Straus 2008) forms the basis of chapter 5. I am grateful to Routledge and to the editors of the *Journal of Musicology* for their permission to reprint parts of those essays here.

During the long period of writing this book, I have had the benefit of guidance from the members of a doctoral seminar on Disability Studies in the Humanities I taught at the CUNY Graduate Center in 2008 and from groups of faculty and graduate students at Rutgers University, the University of Chicago, and Princeton University where I gave presentations. Most recently, in January 2010, I had the privilege of participating in the CUNY Symposium on Music and Disability, and those lively few days gave me much to think about.

A number of people read portions of this book at various times, and I am deeply grateful to all of them for their valuable advice: H-Dirksen Bauman, Licia Carlson, Lennard Davis, Rosemarie Garland-Thomson, Nancy Garniez, Jeff Gillespie, Sally Goldfarb, Dave Headlam, Stefan Honisch (who suggested the title for this book), Blake Howe, Brian Hyer, Stephanie Jensen-Moulton, Simi Linton, Bruce Quaglia, Julia Rodas, Julie Singer, Laurie Stras, Martha Straus, and Tammie Willis. I am also grateful to the editorial team at Oxford University Press, especially Suzanne Ryan, who believed in this project from the very beginning and sustained it throughout.

Among all those who have shaped this book, my deepest intellectual debts are owed to Rosemarie Garland-Thomson. Her book, *Extraordinary Bodies: Figuring Physical Disability in American Culture and Literature (1997)*, was a threshold event in the history of Disability Studies, announcing a new intellectual maturity and sophistication and asserting disability, along with gender, class, and ethnicity, as a fundamental category of cultural analysis. Through that and subsequent works, as well as extended conversations, she opened up to me a world of possibilities and for the past ten years has been an invaluable, generous mentor and guide, and a shining example of politically engaged scholarship.

My son, Michael, is the ultimate source of this intellectual endeavor. My life with him has led me to think about music in a different way, and the way I have come to think about music has in turn influenced my relationship with him. He and his younger brother, Adam, have provided love, support, and welcome distraction without which no intellectual project, and no life, can thrive. Finally, as in my previous books, I acknowledge with deepest admiration, gratitude, and love my peerless partner, Sally Goldfarb.

Extraordinary Measures

INTRODUCTION

D isability is a pervasive and permanent aspect of the human condition: most of us have been, are now, or (as we age) will be people with disabilities.[1] Disability may at first appear inescapably, solidly real—a medically, scientifically, biologically verifiable defect in mind or body. But despite its undeniable material reality, disability is also shaped and given meaning by culture. Attitudes toward disability vary with time and place and so, therefore, does the lived reality of disability. Even the sorts of conditions that are considered disabilities change with time and place. This is particularly evident in the psychiatric or cognitive domain. Some disabilities that were once felt as entirely real exist no longer (e.g., hysteria, neurasthenia, fugue, or nostalgia—all once legitimate medical diagnoses), whereas others that never existed before as distinct entities now seem all too pervasively real (e.g., attention deficit disorder or autism).[2] Even in the physical realm, disabilities come and go, partly under the influence of medical science and partly under the influence of culture (e.g., anorexia, erectile dysfunction, or obesity, now often discussed as a

---

1. The Americans With Disabilities Act (ADA) of 1990 defines *disability* as "a physical or mental impairment that substantially limits one or more major life activities." Using a closely related definition, the U.S. Census of 2000 identifies approximately 50 million Americans over the age of 5 (more than 15% of the population) as people with disabilities. The World Health Organization (WHO) defines an "impairment" as "any loss or abnormality of psychological, physiological, or anatomical structure or function" and a "disability" as "any restriction or lack (resulting from an impairment) of ability to perform an activity in the manner or with the range considered normal for a human being." Under this definition, the WHO estimated in 1980 that 6–7 percent of the world's population (roughly 245 million people) is disabled. Both the ADA and WHO definitions are primarily functional—people are understood as disabled if they are unable to do certain things. Neither definition is concerned with the origin of the disability, which may be congenital or acquired through trauma, disease, or in any other way.

2. See Hacking (1998, 8) for a penetrating discussion of "transient mental illnesses," especially "fugue" (i.e., "undertaking strange and unexpected trips, often in states of obscured consciousness").

medical epidemic). In short, disability is both a material reality and a cultural creation with a long and interesting history.[3]

Disability has recently become a subject for study among scholars in the humanities and social sciences. The newly emerged field of Disability Studies offers a sociopolitical analysis of disability, focusing on social and cultural constructions of the meaning of disability, and shifting our attention from biology (the proper study for science and medicine) to culture (the proper study for humanists).[4] Like gender, disability has a self-evident physical, biological basis: blindness, deafness, paraplegia, and Down syndrome, for example, are objective, factual matters. But, also like gender, the physical, biological facts of disability are endowed with meaning by the elaborate interpretive networks created within particular societies and cultures.[5] And just as feminist theory distinguishes sex from gender, and critical race theory distinguishes race from ethnicity, Disability Studies usually distinguishes "impairment" (an underlying biological or medical condition) from "disability" (the meanings conferred on impairment by social and cultural construction).[6] Disability is

---

3. It would be hard to find a more vivid expression of the idea that disability has a strong cultural component, and is thus subject to changes in fashion, than that offered in a letter by Jane Austen: "What is become of all the shyness in the world? Moral as well as natural diseases disappear in the progress of time, and new ones take their place. Shyness and the sweating sickness have given way to confidence and paralytic complaints." Letter to her sister Cassandra, February 8, 1807.

4. As Garland-Thomson (1997a, 7) argues,

> The meanings attributed to extraordinary bodies reside not in inherent physical flaws, but in social relationships in which one group is legitimated by possessing valued physical characteristics and maintains its ascendancy and its self-identity by systematically imposing the role of cultural or corporeal inferiority on others. Representation thus simultaneously buttresses an embodied version of normative identity and shapes a narrative of corporeal difference that excludes those whose bodies or behaviors do not conform.

Likewise, see Longmore (2003).

5. A central trend in Disability Studies is the effort to disengage disability from a medical model that conceives of disability as a pathology of individual bodies.

> The medicalization of disability casts human variation as deviance from the norm, as pathological condition, as deficit, and, significantly, as an individual burden and personal tragedy. Society, in agreeing to assign medical meaning to disability, colludes to keep the issue within the purview of the medical establishment, to keep it a personal matter and "treat" the condition and the person with the condition rather than "treating" the social processes and policies that construct disabled people's lives. The disability studies' and disability rights movement's position is critical of the domination of the medical definition and views it as a major stumbling block to the reinterpretation of disability as a political category and to the social changes that could follow such a shift (Linton 1998, 11–12).

Likewise, see Longmore and Umansky (2001).

6. As Thomas and Corker summarize the distinction, "Impairments make up the material prerequisite, or substantive premise, for the social enactment of disability" (Thomas and Corker 2002, 20). Likewise, Davis (2002, 12, 41) observes that,

---

simultaneously real, tangible, and physical, yet also an imaginative creation whose purpose is to make sense of the diversity of human morphology, capability, and behavior.

Over the past 300 years, people in the West have thought about disability in four ways: 1) disability as an affliction, permanent and indelible; 2) disability as afflatus (defined as divine inspiration), a mark of transcendent vision; 3) disability as a medical defect, a bodily pathology to be overcome through individual effort; and 4) disability as a personal, cultural, and social identity, to be affirmatively claimed. To some extent, these four models emerge in chronological sequence, but in messy reality they have coexisted and are interrelated in various ways.

In the first model, disability is conceived as a sign of divine disfavor, a punishment by God, and thus the outward mark of an inward moral failing.[7] This was the prevailing pre-Enlightenment view of disability. Although to some extent

---

> Impairment is the physical fact of lacking an arm or a leg. Disability is the social process that turns an impairment into a negative by creating barriers to access.... An impairment involves a loss or diminution of sight, hearing, mobility, mental ability, and so on. But an impairment only becomes a disability when the ambient society creates environments with barriers —affective, sensory, cognitive, or architectural.

This distinction is contested within Disability Studies, in recognition of the contingent, historically inflected, and permeable boundary between the categories. According to Corker and French (1999, 2),

> Social model theory rests on the distinction between disability, which is socially created, and impairment, which is referred to as a physical attribute of the body. In this sense it establishes a paradigm for disabled people which is equivalent to those of sex/gender and race/ethnicity. However, though it is a ground-breaking concept, and one which has provided tremendous political impetus for disabled people, we feel that because the distinction between disability and impairment is presented as a dualism or dichotomy—one part of which (disability) tends to be valorized and the other part (impairment) marginalized or silenced—social model theory, itself, produces and embodies distinctions of value and power.

For a vigorous critique of the impairment/disability distinction, and the social model of disability it undergirds, see Shakespeare (2006, 35): "Impairment is always already social, while disability is almost always intertwined with impairment effects." Likewise, see Scully (2008). Nonetheless, I see the impairment/disability distinction as a useful starting point, a strategic rhetorical move that permits people to begin to focus attention on the social and cultural construction of disability.

7. As Winzer (1997, 76) summarizes,

> In the thousands of years of human existence before 1800, life for most exceptional people appears to have been a series of unmitigated hardships. The great majority of disabled persons had no occupation, no source of income, limited social interaction, and little religious comfort. Conspicuously abnormal persons were surrounded by superstition, myth, and fatalism—especially fatalism. Their lives were severely limited by widely held beliefs and superstitions that justified the pervasive prejudice and callous treatment. Individuals seen as different were destroyed, exorcised, ignored, exiled, exploited—or set apart because some were even considered divine.

supplanted by a medicalized understanding of disability, the moralistic view persists.[8] Think, for example, of the deformed crones of fairy tales, of Ahab in *Moby Dick,* of the title character in Verdi's *Rigoletto*—in each case the physical deformity is a symbol of inner evil. At the present moment, AIDS, addiction, and obesity—and other widely occurring variations in human morphology, behavior, and ability—are often thought of as emblems of character flaws and immorality, the outward manifestations of a contemptible lack of self-control.

In the second model, one with ancient roots but particularly characteristic of the nineteenth century, disability is conceived as a sign of divine inspiration. Madness has long been associated in the popular imagination with creative genius. In a similar fashion, Homer's blindness and Beethoven's deafness have been taken as external signs of an enhanced interiority, a more profound understanding: Homer sees and Beethoven hears more than those with merely normal vision and hearing. In this view, the disability is transcended, left behind as an external marker for a spirit that rises above it. In relation to the first model, disability is still understood as having its source in the divine, but now as afflatus rather than affliction. In relation to the third model, the disability is not overcome through personal struggle, but simply transcended.

A third way of thinking about disability, a way that has been prevalent in the West since around 1800, is a medical model that defines disability as a pathology or defect that resides inside an individual body or mind.[9] These pathologies and defects can be remediated or even cured through medical intervention and personal effort. More broadly, the medical model of disability is an expression of what Garland-Thomson calls "the cultural logic of euthanasia": disabled bodies should either be rehabilitated (i.e., normalized) or eliminated (either by being sequestered from sight in homes or institutions or by being allowed or encouraged to die).[10] Although the medical model is itself historically contingent, changing with evolving

8. Susan Sontag has traced the moralizing responses to tuberculosis and cancer, diseases that have been understood as signs of personal deficiencies (Sontag 1978).

9. Deutsch (2002, 198) locates the emergence of this new conceptualization of disability a bit earlier, in the mid-eighteenth century:

> Suspended between two narrative constructions of the disabled individual, eighteenth-century paradigms of disability existed in formative relation to the concept of individuality. The earlier paradigm viewed disability as a largely visual sign of deserved divine punishment for moral failings, while the modern paradigm conceived of disability as ineffable identity in the familiar narrative terms we now recognize: a vehicle to a proof of inner worth, an obstacle to be heroically conquered by a randomly afflicted individual.

10. See Garland-Thomson (2004a, 779–80):

> This logic has produced conflicting, yet complementary, sets of practices and ideologies that American culture directs at what we think of broadly as disability. Such thinking draws a sharp distinction between disabled bodies imagined as redeemable and others considered disposable. One approach would rehabilitate disabled bodies; the other would eliminate them. I am positing the cultural logic of euthanasia broadly, not simply as ending a life for reasons of "mercy" or eliminating a group targeted as inferior or flawed—such as people with *spina bifida* or "mental retardation"—but as an umbrella concept, a mode of thought manifest in particular notions of choice, control,

medical concepts and practices, it is fundamentally characterized by its adherence to what Scully (2008, 3) calls "the deficit/repair paradigm."[11]

The medical model of disability, like the cultural logic of euthanasia, depends on a fundamental distinction between the normal and the abnormal. The term "normal," along with its cognates (abnormal, norm, normative, normalize), emerged in all of the European languages around 1830. These terms and concepts were brought into being by the new science of statistics, a form of social control in which populations are sorted and evaluated according to various human traits, and normed under the familiar bell-shaped curve, with deviants relegated to the margins. Previously disability had been constructed as monstrosity in opposition to the natural, whereas now disability was to be constructed in accordance with a medical model, that is, as an abnormality defined in opposition to the statistical norm.[12] Instead of being a mark of divine disfavor or inspiration, disability came to be seen as a deviation from a normative standard and thus subject to possible remediation: the normal could be normalized.[13]

This new concept of disability—as an abnormality that might be normalized—coincides with the emergence of institutions and professions that have as their goal

---

happiness, and suffering that underpin a wide range of practices and perceptions. Our culture encodes the logic of euthanasia in its celebration of concepts such as curing, repairing, or improving disabled bodies through procedures as diverse as reconstructive and aesthetic surgery, medication, technology, gene therapy, and faith healing. At the same time, this logic supports eradicating disabled bodies through practices directed at individuals—such as assisted suicide, mercy killing, and withholding nourishment—and those directed at certain groups deemed inferior—such as selective abortion, sterilization, euthanasia, eugenics, and institutionalization.

11. As Scully (2008, 23) amplifies,

There is more than one way of modeling disability in medical terms, in line with the methodological diversity of medicine itself. Broadly, the key feature of a medicalized view is that disability is a nominative pathology: a defect or deficit located in an individual. What counts as defect or deficit is determined by reference to a norm of physical or mental structure and function. The parameters of the norm are given by biomedical science, which since the eighteenth century has increasingly been concerned with quantifying deviation. So from a medicalized perspective, disability is an abnormality of form or function, the cause of which lies in the biology of the individual.

12. On the history of the normal in relation to the medical model of disability, see Baynton (2001) and Davis (1995, 1997a).

13. Baynton (2001, 35) suggests that

The metaphor of the natural versus the monstrous was a fundamental way of constructing social reality in [Edmund] Burke's time. By the late nineteenth and early twentieth centuries, however, the concept of the natural was to a great extent displaced or subsumed by the concept of normality.... The natural and the normal both are ways of establishing the universal, unquestionable good and right. Both are also ways of establishing social hierarchies that justify the denial of legitimacy and certain rights to individuals or groups. Both are constituted in large part by being set in opposition to culturally variable notions of disability—just as the natural was meaningful in relation to the monstrous and the deformed, so are the cultural meanings of the normal produced in tandem with disability.

the remediation of disability.[14] The period around 1800 saw a sudden flowering of facilities for the training and education of the blind and the deaf.[15] People with disabilities thus emerge as a distinct class, and medically oriented institutions and professions emerge to assist them.[16]

14. Stiker (2000, 102) identifies the close of the eighteenth century as the moment when "the idea of formally organizing the disabled and returning them to the level of others makes its entry into history, along with ideas for appropriate technologies and specialized institutions...In short, there was a complete new concern: for *education* and the *rehabilitation of the disabled*" (italics in the original). These new institutions were designed "to offset the objective obstacles that hindered access to a personal and social life. It was no longer a question of simply gathering the disabled together, or even of putting them to work as less than able-bodied. The objective was rather to provide entry to the common cultural and social heritage of their fellow citizens" (107).

15. On institutions for the blind, see Phillips (2004, 18, 27):

> Between 1780 and 1820 establishments were set up across Europe which for the first time sought to educate the blind and train them for work. In France in 1784, in England and Scotland during the 1790s, and shortly afterwards in Austria, Prussia, Holland and elsewhere, enterprises were begun, claiming some kind of educational purpose.... The creation of the blind asylum may be conceived in terms of four propositions—which its founders were required to make to themselves and to others. The first designated the blind as a class with distinctive physical and behavioral characteristics. The second asserted that their condition could be improved by a form of training adapted to these characteristics. The third pronounced the ability to engage in productive work as the principal goal of such training. The fourth identified a formalized, rule-governed institution as the most appropriate means of furnishing it.

> On the history of deaf people and the institutions created to educate them, see Lane (1984). The first public educational institution for deaf people was founded in Paris in 1771 by Abbé Charles Michel de l'Épée. In the subsequent two decades, similar schools, modeled on l'Épée's, were founded throughout Europe, including Bordeaux, Karlsruhe, Prague, Munich, Freising, Linz, and, notably, Beethoven's Vienna.

>> Although the work of l'Épée and his successors did indeed establish for all to see that people who were deaf could be educated to participate creatively in the intellectual, vocational, and artistic realms of social life, these educators also laid the ground for the effective medicalization of deafness and for the entry of deaf people into the ranks of the "disabled" (Branson and Miller 2002, 106).

16. And, in the process, to sequester and control them. The institutions and professions that exist to serve and care for people with disabilities are active participants in the cultural construction of disability—their own existence and longevity depend on it. This is one of the central insights of Michel Foucault—see, for example, Foucault (1978).

> Foucault designates the disciplinary exposé of sexual abnormality and deviance as an addictive professional pleasure that both ensures the longevity of the profession itself and assures the insertion of patients with a determinate catalog of perversions. Disability Studies critiques a similar history of professional parasitism. Disabled communities traditionally have been defined through scientific narratives about aberrancies and physiological dysfunctions that in turn further sustain the need for the professional discourses that define them (Mitchell and Snyder 1997, 25).

Within the past thirty years, a fourth way of thinking about disability has emerged as an alternative to the medical model. Accompanying the political Disability Rights movement, the new interdisciplinary field of Disability Studies understands disability not as a mark of divine disfavor or inspiration nor as a medical pathology but rather as a social and cultural construction. Within this new social model, disability is understood as an aspect of the diversity of human morphology, capability, and behavior: a difference, not a deficit. A new generation of disability activists has begun to "claim disability" as a positive political and cultural identity.[17] In Scully's (2008, 4) memorable phrase, disability has "migrated from pathology to ontology." In an earlier period, and continuing to this day, medical professionals have staked their claim to control people with disabilities, to normalize them, and to represent them to the outside world. Recently, we have begun to see politically aware people with disabilities demanding the right to represent themselves, and explicitly rejecting regimes of normalization.

In this book, disability will be defined as any *culturally stigmatized bodily difference*.[18] By "difference," I refer to deviation from whatever is understood as normal at a particular time and place. As with gender, race, and sexual orientation,

17. The term and concept of "claiming disability" are developed in Simi Linton's (1998) book of that title. For a recent assertion of this central contention of Disability Studies, see Siebers (2008, 3–4):

> While seen historically as a matter for medical intervention, disability has been described more recently in Disability Studies as a minority identity that must be addressed not as personal misfortune or individual defect but as the product of a disabling social and built environment. Tired of discrimination and claiming disability as a positive identity, people with disabilities insist on the pertinence of disability to the human condition, on the value of disability as a form of diversity, and on the power of disability as a critical concept for thinking about human identity in general.... The medical model defines disability as an individual defect lodged in the person, a defect that must be cured or eliminated if the person is to achieve full capacity as a human being.... Unlike the medical approach, the emerging field of Disability Studies defines disability not as an individual defect but as the product of social injustice, one that requires not the cure or elimination of the defective person but significant changes in the social and built environment.... Disability is not a physical or mental defect but a cultural and minority identity. To call disability an identity is to recognize that it is not a biological or natural property but an elastic social category both subject to social control and capable of effecting social change.

18. A related definition that focuses on concepts of normality and deviation uses the term disability to designate "cognitive and physical conditions that deviate from normative ideas of mental ability and physiological function" (Mitchell and Snyder 1997, 2). See also Garland-Thomson (2004b, 76–77) who proposes

> a broad understanding of disability as a pervasive cultural system that stigmatizes certain kinds of bodily variations.... The informing premise of feminist disability theory is that disability, like femaleness, it not a natural state of corporeal inferiority, inadequacy, excess or a stroke of misfortune. Rather, disability is a culturally fabricated narrative of the body, similar to what we understand as the fictions of race and gender. The disability/ability system produces subjects by differentiating and marking bodies.

the construction of disability involves the opposition of a normative standard (e.g., male, white, straight, able-bodied) and a deviant Other (e.g., female, non-white, gay, disabled). Indeed, femaleness, non-whiteness, and gayness can all be understood as forms of disability, and that is how they have often been described historically.[19] In this sense, disability is the "master trope of human disqualification," the fundamental form of deviant Otherness of which gender, race, and sexual orientation are specific manifestations.[20] By "bodily," I refer to the full range of physical and mental differences to which the human body is subject, whether congenital or acquired, including physical and mental illnesses or dis-

Compared to the ADA and WHO definitions discussed above, the definition adopted here, as well as those of Mitchell and Snyder and Garland-Thomson, are less pragmatic in orientation (bodily or mental function) and more concerned with culturally constructed deviation from contextual norms.

19. With regard to gender, for example, a formulation with its roots in Aristotle defines the female body as a "monstrosity," both deviant and inferior with respect to the male body. As Garland-Thomson (1997b, 280) observes:

> More significant than his simple conflation of disability and femaleness is that Aristotle reveals the source from which all otherness arises: the concept of a normative, "generic type" against which all corporeal variation is measured and found to be different, derivative, inferior, and insufficient. Not only does this definition of the female as a "mutilated male" inform later versions of woman as a diminished man, but it arranges somatic diversity into a hierarchy of value that assigns plenitude to some bodies and lack to others based on their configurations. Furthermore, by focusing on defining femaleness as deviant rather than the maleness he assumes to be essential, Aristotle also initiates the discursive practice of marking what is deemed aberrant while concealing the position of privilege by asserting its normativeness. Thus we witness perhaps the originary operation of the logic which has become so familiar in discussions of gender, race, or disability: male, white, or able-bodied superiority is naturalized, remaining undisputed and obscured by the ostensible problem of female, black, or disabled deviance.

Within Disability Studies, there is extensive literature on the relationship of disability to gender, race, and sexuality. See, for example, the essays collected in Smith and Hutchison (2004), as well as Wendell (1996, 1997), LaCom (1997), Baynton (2001), and McRuer (2002).

20. Scholars of gender, race, and sexuality have often sought to distance themselves from the historical stigma of disability:

> As feminist, race, and sexuality studies sought to unmoor their identities from debilitating physical and cognitive associations, they inevitably positioned disability as the "real" limitation from which they must escape.... Biological inferiority had to be exposed as a construction of discursive power. Formerly denigrated identities are "rescued" by understanding gendered, racial, and sexual differences as textually produced, distancing them from the "real" of physical or cognitive aberrancy projected onto their figures.... For all populations physical and cognitive limitations constitute a baseline of cultural undesirability from which they must dissociate themselves in the quest for civil rights and for a lessening of stigmatization. Consequently, disability has undergone a dual negation—it has been attributed to all "deviant" biologies as a discrediting feature, while also serving as the material marker of inferiority itself. One might think of disability as *the master trope of human disqualification* (Mitchell and Snyder 2000, 2–3; italics added).

eases, temporary or permanent injuries, and a variety of nonnormative bodily characteristics understood as disfiguring. By "stigmatized," I refer to any negative social valuation.[21] Obviously, the value assigned to any particular bodily difference will vary from context to context. Nonnormative bodily features and, as we will see, nonnormative musical features, may be understood as either desirable or disabling, depending upon the context. By "culturally," I embrace a conception of disability as socially and culturally constructed, a historically contingent term the meaning of which varies with time, place, and context. By adopting this broad definition, I suggest that disability affects all people and all of their cultural products, paradoxically ubiquitous and yet also perceived as strange and remarkable.[22]

Until now, disability has not entered much into discussions of music.[23] This is probably because music is blessed and cursed by its nonrepresentational nature and by the forbidding technical vocabulary that has grown up around it: both features have tended to isolate music and discussions of music from larger cultural trends. By using mostly nontechnical language (and providing a Glossary of Musical Terms for the inescapable references to musical harmony and form), I hope to bring disability and music into a dialogue that will be comprehensible to nonmusicians.

21. The classic study in this area is Goffman (1963, 3): "The term stigma will be used to refer to an attribute that is deeply discrediting, but it should be seen that a language of relationships, not attributes, is really needed. An attribute that stigmatizes one type of possessor can confirm the usualness of another, and therefore is neither creditable nor discreditable as a thing in itself."

22. As Garland-Thomson (2009, 19–20) observes,

> Each one of us ineluctably acquires one or more disabilities—naming them variably as illness, disease, injury, old age, failure, dysfunction, or dependence. This inconvenient truth nudges most of us who think of ourselves as able-bodied toward imagining disability as an uncommon visitation that mostly happens to someone else, as a fate somehow elective rather than inevitable. In response, we have refused to see disability. Avowing disability as tragic or shameful, we have hidden away disabled people in asylums, segregated schools, hospitals, and nursing homes. When we ourselves develop disabilities, we often hide them as well, sometimes through semantic sleights-of-hand, sometimes through normalizing medical procedures that erase disability, and sometimes through closeting our condition. This hiding of disability has made it seem unusual or foreign rather than fundamental to our human embodiedness. Rather than accepting disability and accommodating it as an expected part of every life course, we are stunned and alienated when it appears to us in others or ourselves.... The visibly disabled body intrudes on our routine visual landscape and compels our attention, often obscuring the personhood of its bearer.

23. The principal publications to date include Straus (2006a, 2006b, 2008), Lubet (2004), and the essays gathered in Lerner and Straus (2006). See also *Popular Music* 28(3) (2009), a special issue devoted to popular music and disability and *The Review of Disability Studies: An International Journal* 4(1) and 4(2) (2008). There is extensive literature on the use of music as therapy for people with disabilities and on the musical perceptions of people with disabilities. This literature will be surveyed in chapter 8.

This book studies the impact of disability and concepts of disability on composers, performers, and listeners with disabilities, as well as on discourse about music and works of music themselves. In chapter 1, I consider composers with disabilities and the critical reception of their music. I show that when critics and general listeners know that a composer has a certain disability, it sharply inflects their perception of the music, and in certain predictable ways. In chapters 2 through 5, I consider various disability-related narratives as they emerge in selected musical works. Despite its inability to represent the world in the manner of language, music is able to tell stories, and among the stories it tells are stories about disability. Some of these stories are narratives of overcoming—the triumph of the human spirit over adversity—but others are more nuanced tales of accommodation and acceptance of life with a nonnormative body or mind. In chapter 6, I consider several critical and theoretical traditions and examine the role of disability-related metaphors in their constructions of musical meaning. Chapter 7 offers a consideration of performers with disabilities, and shows that their performance of their disabilities and the performance of their music are deeply intertwined. Finally, in chapter 8, I turn my attention the act of listening. In response to an accepted notion of normal hearing, I propose several "disablist hearings," that is, ways of hearing music that are inflected by the experience of disability.

This book focuses exclusively on instrumental music of the Western classical tradition: no vocal music (song or opera), no popular or folk music, no non-Western music. I have restricted the repertoire in this way for three reasons, two of them practical and one theoretical. The first reason, a practical one, is simply a matter of scope: there is and has been too much music in the world to begin to encompass it all in a slender book like this. My failure to speak about music outside the West, or about popular or folk traditions inside and outside the West, or even about texted music in the West, is obviously a serious limitation, but I hope not a fatal one. The second reason, also practical, is that this is the music I know and love best, the music I have studied in my career as a music theorist and musicologist, and the music I have played as a cellist.

The third reason, a theoretical one, has to do with my argument that disability is not so much a medical condition as a culture and a political, social, and personal identity. I contend that such disparate figures as Francesco Landini and Glenn Gould, Ludwig van Beethoven and Hikari Oe, have something in common, namely their experience of disability, and that this links them in a shared culture of disability. At first glance, disability may appear to offer a more porous, unstable identity than those conferred, for example, by gender or race/ethnicity.[24] Indeed, the overarching

24. The heterogeneity of the category is described by Garland-Thomson (1997a, 13–15):

> Disability is an overarching and in some ways artificial category that encompasses congenital and acquired physical differences, mental illness and retardation, chronic and acute illnesses, fatal and progressive diseases, temporary and permanent injuries, and a wide range of bodily characteristics considered disfiguring, such as

concept of disability only came into use around 1800—prior to that, conditions like blindness, deafness, madness, and lameness were considered entirely separate, and did not constitute some shared category.[25] But, as recent postmodern theorizing of gender and race/ethnicity has made clear, those categories are also socially constructed, permeable, and inherently unstable. In that sense, disability confers a social, cultural, and political identity as reliable—and unreliable—as those conferred by gender and race.[26] Throughout this book, then, I will insist on the

---

scars, birthmarks, unusual proportions, or obesity. Even though the prototypical disabled person posited in cultural representations never leaves a wheelchair, is totally blind, or profoundly deaf, most of the approximately forty million American with disabilities have a much more ambiguous relationship to the label. The physical impairments that render someone "disabled" are almost never absolute or static; they are dynamic, contingent conditions affected by many external factors and usually fluctuating over time.... Although categories such as ethnicity, race, and gender are based on shared traits that result in community formation, disabled people seldom consider themselves a group. Little somatic commonality exists among people with different kinds of disabilities because needs and situations are so diverse. A blind person, an epileptic, a paraplegic, a deaf person, and an amputee, for example, have no shared cultural heritage, traditional activities, or common physical experience. Only the shared experience of stigmatization creates commonality.... Unlike the ethnically grouped, but more like gays and lesbians, disabled people are sometimes fundamentally isolated from each other, existing often as aliens within their social units.

Likewise, Scully (2008, 21) observes,

Disability is an organizing idea that has to hold together a daunting variety of body states, some universally agreed to be disabling, and others whose status is more contested: sensory impairments, mobility restrictions, missing or lost limbs, skeletal dysplasias (including restricted growth), morphological anomalies ranging from conjoined twins to extra toes, genetic syndromes with complex phenotypes, cognitive impairments and learning difficulties, mental illnesses, disablement due to chronic illness such as HIV/AIDS or metabolic dysfunction, and neurofunctional disorders. The concept of disability also has to cover impairments with different origins.... and it has to account for the fact that there are people with the *same* bodily variation who disagree on whether they are disabled at all.

25. Scully (2008, 22). For a broad historical perspective on disability in concept and practice, see Braddock and Parish (2001).

26. Identities of this kind, and the essentialism they entail, have been the subject of extensive postmodernist critique. As Davis (2002, 13) summarizes:

The disability movement quite rightly desired to include disability as part of the multicultural quilt. If all the identities were under the same tent, then disability wanted to be part of the academic and cultural solidarity that being of a particular, oppressed minority represented. Yet, within that strong notion of identity and identity politics, a deconstructive worm of thought began its own parasitic life. That worm targeted "essentialism." Essentialists were putatively accused of claiming in a rather simple-minded way that being a woman or an ethnic minority was somehow rooted in the body. That identity was tied to the body, written on the body. Rather, the way out of this reductionist mode was to say that the body and identities around the body were socially constructed and performative.... Social

coherence of disability as a category in an effort to show that music (which includes its composers, performers, listeners, critical traditions, and exemplary works) both reflects and constructs disability.

---

constructionism and performativity seemed to offer the way out of the problem caused by the worm of essentialism, but they also created severe problems in shaping notions of identity. If all identities are socially constructed or performative, is there a core identity there? Is there a there?

Likewise, see Shakespeare (2006, 76): "Disability identify politics has been very powerful, but also contradictory and incoherent. This may derive from the heterogeneity of disabled people's experience."

CHAPTER 1

Composers with Disabilities and the Critical Reception of their Music

MODELING DISABILITY, MODELING MUSIC

The Western classical tradition in music is focused on composers and their works. In contrast to most popular, vernacular, and non-Western traditions, the classical tradition tends to celebrate the artistic achievements of exemplary creative individuals and, insofar as the Western classical tradition coheres, it does so around a canon of master composers and their masterworks.[1]

The canon of Western classical composers is not diverse with regard to race, class, or gender, but it is with regard to disability. Beethoven, of course, comes immediately to mind—he is at the center of the canon, and his deafness is at the center of interpretation of his music, especially his late music. But a moment of reflection calls many others to mind: Landini (blind from a young age); Bach and Handel (both blind in their final years, as was Delius); Smetana, Fauré, Ralph Vaughan Williams, and Ethel Smyth (all deaf in their later years); Schubert (the disabling effects of syphilis), Schumann (madness), Milhaud (mobility impairment), Stravinsky (stroke),

---

1. Taruskin (2005) traces this conception to the end of the eighteenth century, pointing to:

> a new concept of the artistic masterwork—a consummate, inviolable, even sacred musical text that contained and transmitted the permanently valuable achievements of a master creator. Thanks to this new concept, the art of music now possessed artifacts of permanent value like the painter's colored canvas or the architect's solid edifice. And like paintings, stored increasingly in public museums, musical masterworks were now worshiped in public temples of art—that is, in modern concert halls, which took on more and more the aspect of museums (vol. 2, 639).

The ideas of the master composer as individual creative genius and the musical work as an autonomous object of nearly sacred value have been subjected to withering critiques in recent years. They are adopted here as a simple heuristic, a point of departure, a strategic move that will permit me to introduce composers' experience of disability into the conversation.

Copland (Alzheimer's disease)—the list goes on and on.[2] What follows is an exploration of the ways in which disability has affected composers, their work, and especially its critical reception. Composers who are diverse in terms of historical period, nationality, and musical style (not to mention race, class, and gender), are linked by the common critical responses to their music in light of their disabilities.

In the Introduction, I identified four conceptual models of disability: divine affliction, divine afflatus, medical pathology, and cultural identity. Critical response to the music of composers with disabilities is almost invariably shaped by one of these models. Under the first two models, music by disabled composers is understood as marked by disability. In some cases, the music appears to share the stigmatized quality of the body that produced it, and is thus judged as deformed or defective (the music is disabled and therefore bad). In some cases, the music appears to be marked by the composer's disability but in a positive way, and the music is judged as visionary or transcendent (the music is disabled and therefore good).

If the disability is understood as a medical pathology, one that may be overcome through personal effort, the disability may be dismissed as a piquant but irrelevant biographical detail (the music is achieved in spite of the disability). A narrative of overcoming disability emerges in the wake of the medical model, with its emphasis on remediation and cure. This becomes the predominant framework for understanding disability: it is something to be eliminated or normalized in the course of a narrative trajectory toward normal selfhood. Within works of music, the overcoming narrative, beginning with Beethoven, takes the form of vigorously and triumphantly overcoming an obstacle created by a discordant element—this will be the topic of chapter 2. In the present chapter, we will see the narrative of overcoming applied to the lives of composers with disabilities, who will be celebrated for what they achieve in spite of disability. In such a scenario, the composer's disability, having been triumphantly overcome, will be judged irrelevant to the music.

It is my hope that music criticism may yet begin to adopt a politically aware understanding of disability. If so, disability may come to be understood as inscribed in the music as a mark of distinction, reflecting the personal and social identity of its creator. Under the sociocultural model of disability, the critical response to composers with disabilities would focus less on what they did in spite of their disability and more on what their disability enabled them to do. These would not be inspirational tales of the triumph of the human spirit over adversity, which is the most familiar way of framing disability. Instead, they would be about understanding the

2. On Smyth, see Wood (2009). From an exclusively medical perspective, O'Shea (1990) and Neumayr (1994, 1995, 1997) discuss the disabilities of Bach, Handel, Mozart, Beethoven, Paganini, Weber, Rossini, Schubert, Mendelssohn, Schumann, Chopin, Liszt, Grieg, Mahler, Delius, Joplin, Grainger, Gershwin, Bartók, Bizet, Borodin, Brahms, Britten, Debussy, Musorgsky, Rachmaninoff, Shostakovich, Scriabin, Haydn, Hummel, Weber, Smetana, and Tchaikovsky. To these, I would quickly add Maria Teresa von Paradies, William Billings, Gabriel Fauré, Antonio de Cabezon, and Allan Petterson (on this last named, see Gimbel [2010]). There will be no end of a list of this kind.

composers as living with disability and creating through disability in a larger context provided by the history of disability: not an affliction to be suffered, not a mark of divine inspiration, not an obstacle to be overcome (and thus ignored), but a source of creative identity. In reality, there has been virtually no criticism of classical composers that views disability in this way. As a result, in what follows, I will be forced to speculate about what such criticism will look like when it finally begins to appear, and to offer some tentative examples of my own.

BLINDNESS

There is a long association between blindness and music, both in the classical and popular music of the West as well as in other parts of the world. In the common imagination, blind people are compensated for their disability with preternaturally acute hearing as well as prodigious musical gifts.[3] Although this is most likely a romantic myth, it is nonetheless true cross-culturally that blind people are often tracked into musical activities when other ways of earning a living might be foreclosed (Rowden 2009; Lerner 2009). As a result, the association of music and blindness is both ancient and widespread.

Western classical music is preeminently dependent on music notation—composers in the West *write* music. Indeed, much of what is distinctive about Western classical music, including its contrapuntal complexity, is dependent on its being part of a written rather than an oral tradition.[4] Blind composers thus approach the enterprise from a distinctive angle: their relationship to the musical materials is not usually mediated by musical notation. Instead, they necessarily maintain strong

---

3. As Sacks (2007, 161) observes,

> The image of the blind musician or the blind poet has an almost mythic resonance, as if the gods have given the gifts of music or poetry in compensation for the sense they have taken away. Blind musicians and bards have played a special role in many cultures, as wandering minstrels, court performers, religious cantors. For centuries, there was a tradition of blind church organists in Europe. There are many blind musicians, especially (though not exclusively) in the world of gospel, blues, and jazz—Stevie Wonder, Ray Charles, Art Tatum, José Feliciano, Rahsaan Roland Kirk, and Doc Watson are only a few. Many such artists, indeed, have "Blind" added to their names almost as an honorific: Blind Lemon Jefferson, the Blind Boys of Alabama, Blind Willie McTell, Blind Willie Johnson. The channeling of blind people into musical performance is partly a social phenomenon, since the blind were perceived as being cut off from many other occupations. But social forces here are matched by strong internal forces.

4. As Taruskin asserts,

> All of the genres that are treated in this book are literature genres. That is, they are genres that have been disseminated primarily through the medium of writing. The sheer abundance and the generic heterogeneity of the music so disseminated in 'the West' is a truly distinguishing feature—perhaps the West's signal musical distinction (Taruskin 2005, vol. 1, xxiii).

affinities with oral and improvisatory traditions. This can be felt in the practical, concrete ways in which they compose. Sighted composers generally notate their music directly, with pen on paper. Blind composers must engage a collaborator to notate what the composers sings or plays. As a collaborative venture, one that is grounded in actual, concrete musical performance, composition by blind composers has distinctive features.[5]

Conceptions of blindness are closely aligned with more general conceptions of disability. In the pre-Enlightenment view, blindness was associated with divinity, either as a divine punishment for transgressions (e.g., Oedipus, Samson) or as a divine afflatus (e.g., Tiresias, Homer).[6] This view remains current: in the popular imagination blindness is still sometimes felt as an outward marker for a higher inner vision. Later understandings of blindness saw it as a medical problem, one that can at least to some extent be moderated with the appropriate medical, surgical, or technological intervention. In this conception, blindness and its effects can be overcome through personal effort and, as a result, need not play a significant role in artistic creation. Critical responses in this vein tend to treat blindness as a piquant personal detail, but one that can be ignored when contemplating the music. The more recent social model of disability, which includes blindness, sees it not as a deficit but rather as a different form of ability. Although this view has flourished in recent years, it has much older roots. Indeed, one finds precursors of it as early as the fourteenth century, in contemporary responses to the medieval-period composer Francesco Landini.

Landini

Landini (ca. 1325–1397), the preeminent composer of *trecento* Florence, was left blind by the smallpox he contracted as a boy. For a very long period, beginning during his lifetime, the critical response to his music was shaped by knowledge of his blindness. In his own time, Landini's blindness was understood as essential to his personal identity and to his music. The relationship between his blindness

---

5. Blind listening has some of the same distinctive features—see chapter 8 for discussion.
6. As Barasch observes,

> The essential characteristic of the blind person's figure, as it appeared to the ancient mind, is his ambiguity.... On the one hand, he is the unfortunate person deprived of sight, the most valuable of senses; on the other, he is often endowed with a mysterious, supernatural ability.... The two sides of the figure, the guilt as well as the prophetic gift, are of sublime origin.... As the guilt of the blind often originates in the contact with the gods, so the unique ability of some of them is also given by the gods.... The gift they have received from the gods is not the power of intercession [as in the later, Christian view]; it is the power to see what will happen, that is, to know the future. It is a sublimated, spiritualized form of vision. What the blind person has lost in his body, the sight of his eyes, he is, at least in some cases, given back in spirit (Barasch 2001, 10–12).

and his music was understood as virtually causal: he is a composer and composes as he does precisely because he is blind.[7]

In contemporary accounts, Landini is generally identified by his first name, Francesco, along with his blindness and sometimes his primary instrument, the portative organ.[8] Some typical descriptions are: "Master Franciscus, Blind Organist of Florence," "The Blind Man of Florence," "blind in his eyes, but illuminated in his soul," "not like a blind man, but more eyed than Argus," and "that Francesco of the organ who sees with his mind more than with his bodily eyes" (Singer 2010). In all of these descriptions, it is assumed both that Landini's blindness is his essential, defining attribute and that his extraordinary musical skill results from it.

The close connection between his blindness and his music is explicit in the only extended contemporary written account, in which Landini's music is understood as a compensation and consolation for his personal tragedy, a light in the presence of darkness.

> None of these [contemporary composers], however—nor, for that matter, any composer of fabled antiquity—can measure up to Francesco, who is still alive, and whom I cannot write about truthfully without some fear of seeming to exaggerate. Francesco was hardly past the middle of his childhood when disaster struck him blind with the smallpox. Music, however, compensated him for his loss with the bright lights of fame and renown. A harsh mischance took away his bodily sight, but his mind's eye was as sharp and acute as an eagle's.... When Francesco had lived for a while in blindness, and was no longer a child, and could understand how miserable it was to be blind, and wanted some solace for the horrors of his everlasting night, he began, as adolescents will, to make up songs—this by the kindness of Heaven, I think, which was preparing in its mercy a consolation for so great a misfortune. When he was a little older still, and had come to perceive music's charm and sweetness, he began to compose, first for voices, then for strings and organ. He made astonishing progress. And then, to everyone's amazement, he took up a number of musical instruments— remember, he had never seen them—as readily as if he could still see. In particular, he began to play the organ, with such great dexterity—always accurately, however—and with such expressiveness that he far surpassed any organist in living memory. All this, I fear, can hardly be set down without some accusation of its having been made up.[9]

Landini's blindness and music are both thus seen in light of the divine, one as an affliction and the other as a mercy. The light of Landini's musical vision is possible only as a response to the darkness of his physical blindness.[10]

7. For this point, and much of the supporting evidence, I am indebted to Singer (2010).

8. A portative organ is one "small enough to be carried or placed on a table, usually with only one set of pipes" (*Harvard Dictionary of Music*).

9. Filippo Villani, *Liber de civitatis Florentiae famisis civibus* (Lives of Illustrious Florentines), reprinted and translated in Wood (1939).

10. As Singer (2010) argues:

The only surviving visual depictions of Landini also make explicit reference to his blindness, and in ways that also engage its divine associations, both negative and positive. In the richly illustrated *Squarcialupi Codex*, which includes most of Landini's surviving musical works, there is a small but beautiful colored drawing of the composer, seated and holding a portative organ, an instrument of which he was an acknowledged master. The drawing dramatizes his blindness, showing him facing to the side, with his one visible eye half closed.[11] The second surviving image of Landini, carved into his tombstone, depicts him with "deep-set, unfocused eyes shrunken into his head" (Singer 2010), again emphasizing his blindness. These representations simultaneously capture a salient biographical fact and link Landini, through a long line of artistic representations, to "blind bards," preeminently Homer, whose blindness is an external mark of a higher vision: the blind person as seer.[12] Both written accounts and visual depictions describe a primary relationship between his blindness and his music, a divine affliction and its merciful compensation.

More recent discussions of Landini, insofar as they talk about his blindness at all, have been more likely to invoke the familiar trope of triumphant overcoming.

> He might have lost his life in one of those dire out-breaks of the plague that made Florence less healthy a city in the 14th century than it is now. Instead the boy Francesco Landini lost his sight as a result of smallpox. Not perhaps the first, but certainly the first famous blind organist in a long line of afflicted musicians leading to Marchal and Walcha in our own day, Landini learnt to triumph over his misfortune and lived a happy and active life, his darkness shedding light on the glorious name of his native city (Stevens 1961, 90).

> [Landini's blindness] may have been the driving force behind his creative activity (and seems to have been regarded by his contemporaries as such). Landini's blindness does not simply heighten the novelty of his situation; his fame derives not from his lack of eyesight, but from the remarkable skill to whose development his blindness was fundamental.

11. I am indebted to Stone (2009) for this interpretation.

12. As Barasch summarizes,

> For some figures blindness may be the external appearance that conceals a mysterious, numinous interior. There is only one type of the sightless—the blind seer or bard—to whom both highly educated authors and popular audiences in antiquity ascribed such a hidden nature. Yet this type, rare as it is, made a profound and lasting impact on the culture of the classical world, and made the blind seer's numinous nature an important component in the image of blindness. [The blind seer] is endowed with the gift of supernatural vision...knowledge that goes beyond the reach of humanity...the uncanny ability to communicate with the world beyond us...an inward vision... seeing with an inner eye (Barasch 2001, 28–29).

According to Stone (2009), the depictions of Landini as blind act as an apparently authentic guarantor of biographical accuracy and immediacy.

Once the disability has been overcome, it need be mentioned no further, for it has no bearing on the music. Indeed, most current scholarship on Landini mentions his blindness only in passing, as an interesting but insignificant personal detail. Where once it was understood as essential, now it is understood as irrelevant to his music.

Yet I think it might be productive to think again about Landini's blindness in relation to his music, and it might be best to begin by thinking about how his music was actually, physically composed. In Landini's time, the late medieval period, musical composition generally involved memory and improvisation. Composers did not jot down musical sketches, then notate successive versions of a musical work, leading to a final score from which individual vocal or instrumental parts could be extracted—that is the procedure of composers from later periods. Rather, composition routinely took place in the memory, in interaction with vocal or instrumental improvisation.[13] At some point, the work would be notated, either by the composer or by a scribe working at the composer's behest. Landini was famous both for his prodigious memory and for his skill as an improviser and, according to contemporary observers, his abilities in both areas were enhanced by his blindness.[14] Indeed, one might say that his blindness enabled him to do more successfully the crucial things that all composers of his day were expected to do. In all of this, Landini operated with relative independence from music notation.

Landini shares his reliance on improvisation and prodigious memory, rather than musical notation, not only with his contemporaries but also with blind musicians throughout the long tradition of blind music-making. These features of "blind listening"—one of the subjects of chapter 8—bind Landini to the community of blind musicians and more broadly to the community of disabled musicians. In thinking about Landini in this way, we are engaging the recent conception of disability as difference, not deficit, focusing not on what Landini was able to do in spite of his blindness, or in triumph over his blindness, but rather on what his blindness enabled him to do. We are accepting that his blindness lies at the core of his artistic achievement. This way of thinking is not reflected in most current scholarship on Landini. Ironically, readmitting blindness as a positive artistic resource and exploring its impact on the music would bring us closer to the conception of Landini held by his contemporaries.[15]

13. On the role of memory in medieval art and music, see Busse-Berger (2005) and Carruthers (2002).

14. As Ellinwood observes,

> If we may judge by the preponderance of his known works (over a third of the extant Italian fourteenth-century music is by him), Landini's compositions must have been popular during his lifetime. Yet his chief glory, like that of many more recent composers, appears to have come from skill as a virtuoso—with him, as an organist. Blindness and the prodigious memory that often accompanies this handicap only served to increase men's admiration for what must have been remarkable skill at improvisation (Ellinwood 1936, 192).

15. As Singer (2010) observes,

Delius

Although Frederick Delius is a much more contemporary figure than Landini (Delius died in 1934), his blindness has provoked similar critical responses to his music. For some, Delius's blindness is an outward mark of a transcendent inner vision and the music takes on an ineffable, other-worldly quality. In a related vein, some critics think of Delius's music as a tale of affliction suffered and over-come—an inspirational story of the triumph of the human spirit over adversity. A countervailing view is that Delius's blindness has no significant impact on his music—the music he wrote before and after he became blind does not differ in any important way. All of these responses to Delius closely track the critical response to Landini.

In addition to these, the critical literature on Delius contains one additional thread: many consider Delius's late music, written when he was blind, to be decid-edly inferior to the earlier music. In this view, the blindness does affect the music, not as a sign of transcendent inner vision, but rather as a stigmatizing mark of its artistic deficiencies: the music is defective just as Delius's body is defective.

Delius was born in 1862 to German parents living in England. Although he is generally thought of as an English composer (and most of the critical literature on the composer comes from that country), he spent most of his life living elsewhere, including a long, final phase in France. He contracted syphilis at some point, prob-ably in 1895, and in its tertiary phase, it led to a variety of physical difficulties, including paralysis of his hands and, by 1922, blindness. His physical condition seemed to preclude composition, but the arrival on the scene of a young musician, Eric Fenby, to serve as his amanuensis, permitted a late flowering of compositional activity. Working collaboratively with Fenby, Delius was able to complete some ear-lier works (e.g., *Cynara* and *A Late Lark*, both for voice and orchestra), salvage some earlier music that had been discarded (e.g., *A Song of Summer, Idyll*), and produce some significant new music, most conspicuously the *Songs of Farewell* for double chorus and orchestra.

The critical response to this body of music is shaped by knowledge of Delius's physical condition, especially his blindness. The familiar critical trope of the blind artist as seer creeps into many accounts:

Landini exemplifies musical excellence in theory and practice alike, as he is a vir-tuoso in both abstract intellectual reflection and in performance.... Landini repre-sents for us the meeting-point of theoretical reflections on the link between blindness and intellectual activity, and the actual production that is its end result. In the abstract, blindness opens the eyes of the mind, as Petrarch would have it, and in prac-tice, according to popular lore, it enhances musical ability. Blindness is thus a physical condition that actuates its own negation (through compensation), giving rise to new intellectual and practical abilities.

Extraordinary Measures

While I was sitting in the garden one evening with Delius, the declining rays of the sun were falling upon a border in such a way that the flowers seemed to have become more ethereal than real. I remarked to him that I wished that he could see them at the moment. I upbraided myself for the tactless remark as soon as it was out of my mouth. I had no need to do so, for he replied that he had no regret that he could no longer see them, for he might be disappointed if he could. They might, he said, be less beautiful than they were in the sight of his imagination. I treasure that evening and that reply as my most pleasant memory of him. Flowers made translucent by the rays of the setting sun. Blindness made translucent by the light of imagination (Oyler 1972, 447).

I recalled his face as it had been when I first knew him—the face of a distinguished technician, severe but debonair. I contrasted my memory of that face with the face I saw before me now. That face had been handsome; this was beautiful. Two qualities were common to both: extreme sensibility and a signal serenity. One of these had increased and, in so doing, now revealed, while the evening light shone upon apparent darkness and disorder, the meaning of the solitary pilgrimage soon to be accomplished. I pondered that serenity and decided it was due to his "devotion to something afar from the sphere of our sorrows," namely beauty (Nichols 1976, 113).

All through his self-guided life he was blind to what he was doing, blind in the highest sense of the word, directing his untiring energy to the worship of Pure Beauty as a supreme end in itself (Fenby 1981, 177).

Despite these evocative descriptions, however, few critics actually ascribe these transcendent features to the music itself. Instead, the critics are sharply divided into two camps: those who think that the music represents a triumph over disability and those who think it is marred by disability. Anthony Payne is in the triumphalist camp:

It is fairly obvious that his physical deterioration was making composition more and more difficult, and in 1925 work stopped altogether. Aged sixty-three, shortly to become a hopeless paralytic, blind, and suffering from racking muscular spasms, his contemporaries can be forgiven for thinking that the spring had dried up permanently. But Delius had one last card up his sleeve; with the help of Eric Fenby, who offered his services as amanuensis, he came back to life. First, there was the dictation of revisions of old scores for the 1929 Delius Festival, and later, with the rapport completely established, the achievement of a full-length masterpiece, *Songs of Farewell* (1930–1932), which, although rich in chromaticism, is, nevertheless, the least luxurious of his choral works. It is bracing and exultant with, in places, an almost Holstian clarity. The powerful last testament of *Songs of Farewell* must finally give the lie to those who, with limited knowledge of a few of Delius's small nature pieces, smugly over-emphasize his limitations. Rather should they marvel that the same style could have produced such different works as *Songs of Farewell* and *Songs of Sunset*, or *In a Summer Garden* and *North Country Sketches*; that within his limits, Delius achieved such variety (Payne 1961–62, 16).

For others, however, Delius's late music is marred by traces of his disability, not just his blindness and paralysis, but the underlying disease that caused them. Gray (1976) refers to the "unmistakably morbid quality" (143) of the later work compared with the "more virile, energetic, exuberant quality" of the earlier work. (144), and argues,

> Apart from the fact that there is not a shred of material evidence in support of it, I am convinced that the clue to the problem is to be found in the affliction from which Delius suffered, the cause of his blindness, paralysis, and death, and to which it is now possible to refer without giving offense to any living person, namely, syphilis. It is to this source that I attribute the lack of formal balance and critical sense, the technical instability and cloying chromaticism, the phenomenal egocentricity amounting almost to *folie de grandeur* which characterize his later years (Gray 1976, 144).

Without Gray's smug moralizing, other critics have rendered a similar judgment: according to Jefferson (1972, 107), Delius's late music represents "the desperate final outpourings of the crippled composer."

For many of the negative critics, the nature of the collaboration with Fenby is the principal point of contention. Western art and culture have long prized individuality and autonomy: great works of art are supposed to be the product of a single inspired mind. If Delius's late music is really by Fenby, at least in some significant degree, then its value is diminished.

As Fenby describes the nature of the collaboration, it becomes clear that he did indeed play a significant creative role and was an active partner rather than a passive scribe.

> The technique of dictation varied, often considerably, with each work. Much depended on the extent to which Delius had already arranged and sifted in his mind the musical matter of what he was going to say before calling for me to note it down. Sometimes he had no more than the roughest idea of what he wanted until that rough idea had been played over to him at the piano.... [With a solitary exception,] Delius always worked in the music-room, I sitting at the keyboard and playing each dictation for his correction or emendation before writing a note of it into the score. Again and again the work of several days proved to be but a mere stepping-stone to something finer. Delius was never able to think of and retain more than a few bars at a time (Fenby 1981, 131–32).

Sometimes Delius would give very explicit instructions (e.g., "cellos play their low F# for seven beats"), but often his indications were considerably vaguer (e.g., "Now the same thing a half note lower and change the harmony" [Fenby 1981, 149]). The composer Percy Grainger recalls hearing Delius give similarly vague instructions: "Put chords to it like those at the end of the Prelude to *Hassan*.... No, make them sound more hollow. Use more open fifths" (Grainger 1976, 126–27). In such cases, Fenby had to use his own creativity and ingenuity: "When I was not writing during his dictation I was feeling my way at the keyboard, striking every note immediately after he had named it, and anticipating whenever possible what I thought would be the next chord as well as my musical instincts and his verbal directions would allow" (Fenby 1981, 149). This suggests something more like a full collaboration rather than simple dictation, as Fenby uses his own creative instincts effectively to improvise in the style of Delius.

For some critics, the nature of Fenby's collaboration with Delius raised questions of authorship and authenticity: are these works, which bear Delius's name, really by Delius?

> Eric Fenby volunteered to help Delius with his music. He has described in his book *Delius as I Knew Him* how he managed to put on paper what Delius tried to dictate to him. I do not accept his explanation. My opinion is that he made himself so familiar with Delius's music that he guessed the sort of theme that Delius would write himself and that, when he played it, Delius agreed to it. I say this without any musical knowledge whatsoever, but merely because Delius himself confessed to me that he did not know what he had composed and what Eric had! (Oyler 1972, 444).

A more informed judgment, but one that expresses a similar unease about collaborative authorship, comes from Thomas Beecham, a long-time champion and close associate of Delius:

> A short reference must be made to the series of pieces he turned out between 1929 and 1933 in conjunction with Eric Fenby. The only epithet that can be applied to this strangest of collaborations is—heroic. But it would be idle if in our admiration for the remarkable qualities of the two participants we ignored the plain fact that it gives us little of Delius that we did not know before; and even that little does not ring with the sound of unadulterated inspiration. Let us honour it as a noble experiment and leave it at that (Beecham 1959, 217–18).

For Beecham, then, the late music is "adulterated," authorially impure, and thus impossible to judge: it is not the real Delius.[16] And, indeed, artists with disabilities are often required to pass an implicit test of authenticity—the public wants reassurance that someone so obviously impaired could really have produced the work ascribed to him or her.

16. Similar questions of authorial authenticity have arisen in connection with works left incomplete because of the death of composer and later finished by someone else—a kind of posthumous collaboration. Mozart's *Requiem* and Berg's *Lulu* are the most prominent examples.

The positive judgments of Delius's late music have generally claimed that the music is good despite the disability, usually in triumph over it: the disability should be ignored in evaluating the music. The negative judgments of Delius's late music have generally claimed that it is bad because of the disability, either because the bodily defects of the composer have led to defective music, or because the composer's disability has led him to an illegitimate and inauthentic collaboration.

An additional possibility, that the late music is informed by the disability, but in ways that are distinguishing and even desirable, has yet to be explored by Delius's critics. Such an approach might place Delius in relation to other blind composers and musicians, hearing in his music some of the shared values of that community. These include a relative freedom from musical notation, and its implicit theoretical biases, a commitment to improvisation, and the need for assistance and collaboration.

People with disabilities have long understood the need for assistance of all kinds to augment their powers and permit them to function effectively. From this perspective, Delius's collaboration with Fenby, rather than an illegitimate subversion of autonomous authorial individuality instead represents simply the way that people with disabilities often go about their lives—collaboratively and interdependently.[17] A critical perspective on Delius that claimed blindness as a cultural identity would see his collaboration with Fenby, along with their improvisatory way of working, as manifestations of blind musical culture.

DEAFNESS

Beethoven

Music is intimately bound up with the sense of hearing, and a deficiency in that sense is generally understood as particularly problematic for musicians. As Beethoven lamented in the early stages of his progressive deafness,

---

17. With reference to autonomy and interdependence, Siebers (2008, 182) observes,

> A focus on disability provides another perspective by representing human society not as a collection of autonomous beings, some of whom will lose their independence, but as a community of dependent frail bodies that rely on others for survival.... My point is not that disabled persons are dependent because of their individual properties or traits. It is not a matter of understanding disability as weakness but of construing disability as a critical concept that reveals the structure of dependence inherent to all human societies. As finite beings who live under conditions of scarcity, we depend on other human beings not only at those times when our capacities are diminished but each and every day, and even at those moments when we may be at the height of our physical and mental powers.

These issues will be discussed more fully in chapter 8.

It was impossible for me to say to people, "Speak louder, shout, for I am deaf." Ah, how could I possibly admit an infirmity in the one sense which ought to be more perfect in me than others, a sense which I once possessed in the highest perfection, a perfection such as few in my profession enjoy or ever have enjoyed (*Heiligenstadt Testament*, quoted in Jander 2000, 25–26).

Yet a significant number of composers have been deaf in one degree or another and have learned to function with and through their deafness. Beethoven of course is preeminent among these, as he is preeminent within the canon of Western classical music.[18]

In many ways, Beethoven's life and work epitomize what was then a new recuperative model of disability. Only a few years before Beethoven began to go deaf, one of the first schools for the deaf was founded a few miles from his home in Vienna, one of many such schools springing up throughout Western Europe. These schools embodied the then-new idea that deafness could be remediated and at least partly overcome. This new idea shaped Beethoven's attitude toward his own deafness: throughout his life, he took advantage of every technological innovation to mitigate his deafness, and his works express in a variety of ways his sense that deafness could be overcome.[19]

If the medical model of disability as something to be overcome pervades Beethoven's life and work, the pre-Enlightenment model of disability as divine affliction or afflatus has shaped critical response to Beethoven's music. Critics have long divided Beethoven's music into three periods, and have often observed how closely these are correlated with his experience of deafness: an early, exuberant period before he became aware of his incipient deafness; a "heroic" middle period replete with narratives of overcoming during a time of deepening hearing loss; and a late period of remarkable innovation coincident with increasingly complete deafness.[20]

The critical reception of Beethoven's late period music has undergone dramatic changes over the years, and these changes are closely tied to prevailing attitudes about deafness in general and Beethoven's deafness in particular. During Beethoven's

18. For a summary and critique of the extensive literature on Beethoven's physical and mental health issues, including his deafness, see Davies (2001) and Larkin (1970).

19. The role of deafness in Beethoven's music will be a principal topic of chapter 2.

20. See, for example, Kinderman (2009, 71):

The relationship between Beethoven's deafness and his artistic development is fascinating. Despite his initial fears, and now discredited attempts to characterize his late style as a degeneration resulting from a lack of hearing, his art actually became richer as his hearing declined. Whereas the evolution of his so-called heroic style closely paralleled the personal crisis articulated in his *Heiligenstadt Testament*, the emergence of his late style, or "third period," was marked by the complete erosion of his hearing many years later, around 1818. The parallel between Beethoven's stylistic development and his increasing deafness is more than coincidental, and it has not escaped notice.

lifetime, his late works were seen as artistically inferior and defective, the direct result of his inability to hear (Wallace 1986). A typical response from 1823 refers to

> that deplorable calamity, the greatest that could befall a man of his profession, his extreme deafness, which we are assured is now so great as to amount to a total privation of hearing. Those who visit him are obliged to write down what they have to communicate. To this cause may be traced many of the peculiarities visible in his later compositions (Ayrton 1823, 156).

In the generation immediately after Beethoven's death, critics identified a third period (i.e., the late style) to segregate the apparently defective final works from the healthy ones that came before. Their motivation was quarantine, not celebration. Even more than the earlier music, the final period music was understood as having a specific physical origin in Beethoven's deafness. Critics tamed the problematic late music by finding its origins in physical pathology and segregating it from the rest (Knittel 1995).

Beginning with Wagner, critics continued to segregate the late period music on the basis of Beethoven's deafness, but now in order to valorize rather than pathologize it. As Scott Burnham (2001a, 111) observes,

> Indeed, of all his music, the music of the so-called late period has undergone the biggest transformation in its reception. Many early critics held these works to be the symptoms of illness; the prevailing later view prefers to understand them as the highest testimony to his genius. The decisive turn to this latter view was helped by Wagner's influential monograph of 1870, written for Beethoven's centenary, in which he glorified Beethoven's deafness as a trait of enhanced interiority—the deaf composer forced to listen inwardly.[21]

From a personal affliction, Beethoven's deafness has come to seem a mark of divine inspiration—by cutting Beethoven off from the conventional and the quotidian, deafness enabled him to ascend the spiritual heights. Here the Romantic idea of the creative genius coincides with the pre-Enlightenment conception of disability as a mark of divinity.

Beethoven scholarship may yet come to an understanding of disability as difference, not deficit. In this view, Beethoven's late music would be shown to have taken the form it did not regardless of his deafness, and not in spite of his deafness, and not in triumph over his deafness, but rather because of his deafness. Such a critical approach would bind Beethoven to a larger community of deaf musicians, and find in his late music an expression of the musical values of that community. As will

21. For important elaboration of this idea, see Knittel (1998, 2002).

be discussed in chapter 8, the deaf relationship to music tends to be visual, tactile, and kinaesthetic. Deaf people often prefer to see the sources of the musical sound, to feel the musical vibrations, and to engage music with bodily movement. Furthermore, the deaf relationship to music tends to emphasize inner hearing, via musical notation and silent contemplation. Many of these preferences resonate with features of Beethoven's music that have been widely discussed in the musicological literature, including most obviously its frequent dance-like qualities and its inwardness. An account of Beethoven's late music that "claimed disability" would situate these musical features in relation to the history and culture of deaf music-making.

Smetana

Unlike Beethoven, Smetana went deaf suddenly. In the summer of 1874, at the age of fifty and at the height of his reputation as the central figure in a revitalized Czech musical culture, the syphilis he had contracted in his youth, now in its tertiary stage, produced a variety of impairments that prevented him from ever again hearing normally (Neumayr 1997).

> It is my cruel destiny that I may lose my hearing. In my right ear I hear nothing, and in the left very little. So I am going deaf. This is the state of my health, of which since July I have tried to cure myself. It was in July, the second day, that I noted the higher octaves in my ear were tuned at a different pitch. From time to time I had a rushing noise in my ears as if I was standing near a forceful waterfall. The condition was continuously changing until the end of the month when it became permanent.... For me, this is a tragedy.[22]

In search of a cure, Smetana tried a variety of quack remedies—the best that the medical science of the time had to offer—that increased his misery without restoring his lost hearing.[23] In time, the syphilis led to a variety of mental disturbances and Smetana died in 1884 in the Prague Lunatic Asylum (Large 1970; Katz 1997).[24]

During the first five or so years after the onset of his deafness, Smetana continued to write productively and well. Indeed, several of the works for which he is still best known, including *Ma Vlast* (My Country) were composed during that period. One of the works from that period, the String Quartet No. 1 ("From My Life"), is a

22. Letter to Dr. Cízek, September 5, 1874. Cited in Large 1970, 244.
23. According to Neumayr (1997), these remedies included complete abstention from piano playing and conversation, an "air douche" (i.e., blowing air into his ears through a rubber tube), and a prolonged "smear treatment," in which his whole body was coated with a salve of unknown content (possibly containing mercury), "electrotherapy," and the puncturing of the skin behind his ears with needles.
24. The most complete description of Smetana's medical history is Feldmann (1971).

programmatic piece that traces significant experiences from throughout his life, a sort of musical autobiography, including a representation of his deafness. In the composer's words, the quartet is "a remembrance of my life and the catastrophe of complete deafness."[25] In the final movement, a piercing, sustained note in the highest register represents the tinnitus that was one component of his hearing disorder: "The long insistent note in the finale...is the fateful ringing in my ears of the high-pitched tones which, in 1874, announced the beginning of my deafness. I permitted myself this little joke because it was so disastrous to me."[26]

Despite the sharp turn in Smetana's biography with the onset of his deafness in 1874, in general the literature on Smetana does not refer to any distinctive late-period style. There is no acknowledged radical change in musical style, no shocking innovations, no hermetic introspection as in Beethoven's late style. The String Quartet No. 1 references Smetana's deafness, but does so within a stylistic framework that had not changed much since he had reached his compositional maturity decades earlier.

The last works Smetana wrote, however, when his deafness was nearly total and his mind was increasingly disordered, have posed a problem for critics and listeners. The String Quartet No. 2 is Smetana's last completed work and he intended it as a continuation of the first, as a musical expression of his life with deafness: "This quartet moves forward from where the first one left off, after the catastrophe. It depicts the turmoil of music in a person who has lost his hearing" (quoted in Neumayr 1997, 182).[27] This work has elicited something of the same contradictory critical response that met Beethoven's late works: are its striking formal idiosyncrasies and harmonic innovations evidence of his failing powers or of a new and higher level of creative achievement?[28]

Smetana himself had doubts about the quality of the work:

25. Letter to Srb-Debrnov, February 10, 1879. Cited in Large 1970, 317.
26. Letter to Srb-Debrnov, April 12, 1878. Cited in Large (1970, 318). A more extensive account from a letter to August Kömpel is provided in Neumayr (1997, 176–78):

> I believed I had to portray the beginning of my deafness and I sought to depict it as happens in the finale of the quartet with the E of the first violin stroked four times. For before the onset of my complete deafness for many weeks in the evenings between 6 and 7 o'clock I was always pursued by the strong whistle of the A-flat major chords, A-flat, E-flat, and C, in the highest piccolo key, uninterrupted for a half hour, indeed, often for a whole hour, and there was no way to free myself of it. This happened regularly each day, as it were, as a warning cry for the future! I therefore have tried to portray this horrible catastrophe in my destiny with the high-pitched E in the finale. Therefore the E must be played fortissimo the whole time through.

27. Neumayr's source is not identified.
28. The critical responses are surveyed in Katz (1997).

[T]he quartet is finished except for the finale, but to find a real conclusion with chords and cadences is difficult. At times I get confused, but I no longer have spots before my eyes and the rushing in my ears is less forceful. Alas, I tend to lose my memory when composing so that if a movement is too long I cannot remember the principal melody. If the working out takes some time I forget the qualities of the melody and look on it as if it were the work of a stranger. How weak my memory is! I tend to lose track of ideas, but in spite of this I want to work and perhaps will emerge victorious in my struggle (Large 1970, 376–77).

Many critics have complained about the sectionalized, atomized quality of the musical flow, and they attribute its seeming incoherence to Smetana's declining mental powers. Other critics have simply turned away, apparently embarrassed by the work's deficiencies. As Katz observes, "It is difficult to avoid the conclusion that the quartet has been tainted by its composer's illness and that commentators have refrained from closely examining the quartet either out of pity for a composer who was no longer competent to ply his trade or because, as a product of disease, the quartet must itself be diseased" (Katz 1997, 519).

Counterbalancing this is a strain of critical response that sees in the String Quartet No. 2 a work whose fractured quality is powerfully expressive, and whose unusual form and harmony are well suited to the emotions Smetana was trying to express: in other words, the lived reality of life after a "catastrophe." In this view, the quartet is neither a descent into madness nor a "triumph of spirit" (to refer to the duality suggested in the title of Katz's article). The work does not succumb to deafness and illness, nor does it overcome them. Rather, it is enabled by Smetana's disability to take its distinctive form and sound.

Gabriela Lena Frank

In our own time, disability still strongly inflects the critical response to a composer's music, but that response may reflect changing social and cultural constructions of disability: as attitudes toward disability change, critical response to the music of composers with disabilities changes also. There is an interesting contemporary American composer named Gabriela Lena Frank who grew up with hearing loss at a time of Deaf cultural activism, amid assertions of deafness as an identity rather than a disability. Although Frank is no activist, and does not identify with the Deaf community, her attitude toward her deafness is nonetheless shaped by these larger social forces. Her deafness, she asserts, has served to individuate her, to free her from the necessity of observing the musical conventions that seemed to restrict nondisabled composers:

[My hearing loss] made me feel right from the beginning that I was different. There's a definite music gene floating around in the family. We have perfect pitch, so in some ways

I hear very well. We have very good memories. So these concerts I went to as a little girl, I would come out of the folkloric concerts having memorized all the songs on one hearing. They just stayed with me, and I would replicate them at the piano. We're all pianists, very fast fingers. We can improvise really, really well, and we can mimic styles very quickly. So that has nothing to do with hearing loss. Hearing loss is just volume. From the beginning, I always felt like I was some sort of underdog and that it was OK for me to be unique and different in that way. I didn't need to be so polite in observing rules, and I think that that philosophy has carried through in the multicultural leanings that I've taken with my music, as well (Oteri 2008).

Frank's relationship to music is more visual and more based on sonic vibration than "normal" hearing (this issue will be discussed in greater detail in chapter 8).

[My first piano teacher] would play something, and I would imitate it back. I didn't really hear the piano; I felt the vibrations through the instrument. It's possible I got my perfect pitch that way at that formative time for brain development. Little kids learn languages very quickly and pick up things very quickly. They identified that I needed hearing aids when I was mainstreamed into a regular kindergarten class. My teacher used to work with deaf kids. She was this little Dutch woman, real short, and she had a piano in the class. I was real bossy, and I would grab all the other little kids and sit them down and I'd give them something to do. Then I would improvise along, and I would push their hands a little higher if I wanted to do other things or a little lower. She saw how I used my eyes all the time; I was always watching other people (Oteri 2008).

As mentioned above, Frank is not committed to Deaf rights nor does she identify with the Deaf community (among other things, she reads lips rather than communicating through American Sign Language), but she still claims disability as part of her identity.[29] For her, deafness is not irrelevant, not a curse or an affliction, not a mark of divine inspiration, nor a medical pathology for which she seeks a cure. Instead, it plays a positive, generative role at the core of her musical creativity.

At the present moment (2009), there is nothing whatsoever in the admittedly small critical literature about Frank that refers to her deafness—either the critics are unaware of it or they consider it irrelevant. In her own discussions of deafness, Frank seems ambivalent about the value, for her, of Deaf political awareness and activism—she seems at once dismissive and intrigued. If it should happen that she

---

29. According to Frank, "there is a segment of the deaf community that would consider me like a light-skinned person trying to pass. You know, they're so passionate about deaf identity that they even use deaf with a capital D. Deaf studies has appropriated a lot from women's studies and African-American studies, in terms of looking at their history as a people. It's very, very interesting. But that's not been my experience, so I don't identify with that. My hearing loss has been something so personal that it's not something that I necessarily politicize" (Oteri 2008).

decides to claim her deafness in a public way, she may yet compel her critics to come to terms with it.

MADNESS

The history of madness tracks the history of disability generally and can be likewise described in three large historical phases. The earliest models of madness involved gods and demons: the mind is possessed by suprahuman forces. As with the pre-Enlightenment model of disability generally, this demonic model of madness has great tenacity—it has never been fully supplanted, and continues to flourish in ages of religious fundamentalism, such as our own. During the nineteenth century, this model of madness flourished in a particular way, in the association of madness with creative genius.[30]

With the Enlightenment, madness came to seem a concrete abnormality, a form of illness or disease, lodged within an individual body or mind.[31] As the medical model of mental and emotional distress took hold, there was a proliferation of diagnostic categories. The older theory of humors rooted in organs of the body gave way to a new theory of nerves: mental illnesses (and they now were understood as illnesses) were thought to result from imbalances or other disorders of the nervous system.[32] A set of conditions and behaviors that would previously have been grouped together under the undifferentiated heading of madness, now splintered into a set of amorphous and shifting categories, including hypochondria, nostalgia, neurasthenia, melancholia, and hysteria. These diagnoses may seem quaint and merely metaphorical now, but they were considered technical, medical terms in their day (and it will not be surprising if our own apparently scientific and medical categories of psychiatric

---

30. Burstein (2006) offers a critical account of the large literature on madness and genius in the course of a study of a famously "mad" composer of the nineteenth century, Charles-Valentin Alkan.

31. As Porter (2002, 58) observes,

> Overall, therefore, Cartesian dualism posed an audacious challenge—one with momentous medical consequences for reasoning about madness, since it implied that as consciousness was inherently and definitionally rational, insanity, precisely like regular physical illnesses, must derive from the body, or be a consequence of some very precarious connections in the brain. Safely somatized in this way, it could no longer be regarded as diabolical in origin or as threatening the integrity and salvation of the immortal soul, and became unambiguously a legitimate object of philosophical and medical enquiry.

32. According to Davis (2008, 53),

> This new era in which almost all maladies might be thought of as nervous further expands the reach and grasp of the medical profession into the realm of the new "nervous diseases" while it ramps up the connection between the mind and the body as well....We have moved from demonic possession, to humoral/organ theory, and finally to the matrix of the nervous system.

"illness"—e.g., schizophrenia, autism—suffer a similar historical fate). In the wake of this conceptual shift came the professions and institutions designed to diagnose and remediate, but which also sequester and incarcerate.[33]

In recent years, a new concept of madness has emerged, one that rejects the medical model (i.e., sickness, illness, disease, cure) in favor of an appreciation of the diversity of human embodiments, both mental and physical.[34] Under the banner of slogans like "the dangerous gift" (with reference to bipolar disorder), "neurodiversity" (with reference to autism), and "psychocrip" (an in-your-face reappropriation of a stigmatized category, modeled on "crip" and "queer"), activists are arguing that madness, so long medicalized as "mental illness," may be better understood as part of the natural diversity of human minds, with a claim for acceptance and accommodation rather than normalization and cure. Amid the search for a new, nonmedicalized terminology for people whose outlook and behavior differs significantly from the prevailing standard of normality, the traditional term "madness" is a useful placeholder, and I will continue to use the term here for a wide range of psychiatric or psychological issues.

Schumann

Many canonical composers in the Western classical tradition have had experiences of madness, if that term is defined broadly to include a variety of mental, psychological, or emotional differences, or deviations from the local normative standard. In discussions of music and madness, Robert Schumann is often the first composer who comes to mind. Schumann had a lifetime of experiences of madness, including episodes of deep depression, periods of heightened activity approaching mania, and aural hallucinations. After a suicide attempt in 1854, Schumann asked to be moved to an asylum, where he died two years later.

33. As Porter (2002, 122) summarizes,

> The asylum idea reflected the long-term cultural shift from religion to scientific secularism. In traditional Christendom, it was the distinction between believers and heretics, saints and sinners, which had been crucial—that between the sane and the crazy had counted for little. This changed, and the great divide, since the "age of reason," became that between the rational and the rest, demarcated and enforced at bottom by the asylum walls. The keys of St. Peter had been replaced by the keys of psychiatry. The instituting of the asylum set up a *cordon sanitaire* delineating the "normal" from the "mad," which underlined the Otherhood of the insane and carved out a managerial milieu in which that alienness could be handled.

34. As Davis (2008, 22) observes,

> Contemporary critics of psychiatry, many of whom are or were users of psychiatric services, have tried to call attention to the problematics of the medical model by refusing to call themselves "mental patients," preferring instead to use the term "mental health service users" or "consumers," and eschewing "mental illness" for the less medicalized "mental distress."

During his lifetime and up to the present moment, psychiatrists with an interest in music and musicologists with an interest in psychiatry have attempted to diagnose Schumann. In a remarkable outpouring of the medical model of madness, proposed diagnoses have included "incomplete general paralysis," melancholia, dementia praecox, neurosyphilis, schizo-affective disorder, manic-depressive disorder, schizophrenia, depression, major affective disorder, and borderline personality disorder.[35] In addition to this bewildering array of psychiatric conditions, Schumann also apparently had a variety of physical illnesses with

35. "Incomplete general paralysis" and "melancholia" are both suggested by Franz Richarz, who was the psychiatrist who cared for Schumann in the asylum at Endenich. The term "incomplete general paralysis" may be an oblique reference to syphilis—there is dispute in the literature on this point. "Dementia praecox" is a diagnosis offered by the German neurologist Paul Möbius in 1906. This diagnosis, either under its original name or its later name, schizophrenia, has been taken up by subsequent accounts also. According to Ostwald (1985, 300), Möbius tried "to prove that genius and madness had something in common, namely, a process of 'degeneration,' rooted supposedly in the individual's racial and genetic background." Neurosyphilis, an infection of the brain or spinal chord resulting from untreated syphilis, was proposed in 1906 by Hans Gruhle and is reaffirmed in Sams (1971). "Schizo-affective disorder" is suggested by Sacks (2007), O'Shea (1990), and Ostwald (1985, 304): "An obsessive-compulsive quality of worry and 'nervousness' seems to have been part of some of Schumann's depressive episodes, while a bizarre, schizophrenic-like quality accompanied some of his manic episodes, especially the one leading up to his hospitalization. (The term 'schizo-affective' disorder might be applicable here)." Some of the same sources have argued also for "manic-depressive disorder." "Schizophrenia" is the diagnosis preferred by Neumayr (1995, 360, 362):

> When we incorporate all aspects of Schumann's artistic accomplishments into his medical history, with its variegated palette of symptoms and the on-again, off-again course it ran, then taken in sum, they certainly argue strongly for the presence of a cyclic psychosis, in other words, a manic-depressive disease of some kind....A periodic manic-depressive psychosis whose first manifestation came with the attack in the year 1933. But because many of the ancillary symptoms do not fit with the concept behind this term, we must, I believe, assume the existence of a so-called "composite psychosis," one in which the symptoms of schizophrenia are also evident amid signs of cyclic depression and where, in the case of Schumann, the most likely of the many forms of schizophrenia was the one called periodic catatonia....This form of schizophrenia, with its bipolar process (phases of heightened activity on the one hand and phases of inertia and extreme withdrawal to the point of "wrapping one's self in a cocoon," on the other), best explains Schumann's symptoms.

Neumayr also thinks that "the organic degenerative process affecting Schumann's brain" resulted from "progressive paralysis caused by syphilitic infection" (363). Ostwald (1985, 201, 303) rejects schizophrenia, preferring instead "a major depressive disorder" or "a major affective disorder":

> Schizophrenia is not a diagnosis one can apply to Schumann with a great deal of confidence. His illness in 1844 and 1845 resembles more closely a major depressive disorder, with some paranoid thinking (now unusual in illnesses of this sort) plus alternating agitation and apathy.... The most comprehensive diagnosis for Schumann's psychiatric illness would be a *major affective disorder*. He suffered from severe, recurring depressive episodes.... Schumann also had mood swings in the opposite direction, toward mania, which makes this a "bipolar" type of affective disorder.

potential psychological or emotional consequences, including malaria, tuberculosis, and syphilis.[36] For this constellation of medical issues, both mental and physical, Schumann received the full array of cutting-edge, state-of-the-art treatments, including hydrotherapy (i.e., bathing or swimming), hypnotherapy, magnetism, and bleeding by leeches.[37]

Much of this psychiatric and medical terminology either postdates Schumann or was otherwise unavailable to him. But medical theories based on the nerves were part of his own self-understanding. He (and Clara Schumann, his virtuoso pianist and composer wife) frequently made reference to his nerves and the danger of their overstimulation, with discussions of "nervous sickness," "nervous complaints," and "nervous affliction" (Ostwald 1985; Neumayr 1995). That medicalized framework reflects the encroachment of the medical model of madness during Schumann's own time:

> It is interesting to note that when he returned from Russia with his wife, Schumann stopped applying the term "madness" to himself. He now used the term "illness" almost exclusively. This too reflected a changing philosophy, which had recently spread from France to other European countries. In 1836, Louis-Francois Lelut published a "pathography" in Paris that claimed Socrates was mentally ill and not simply possessed by demons, as had been believed earlier. A similar conclusion about Blaise Pascal appeared in 1846. (Ten years later—the year Schumann died—another French psychiatrist, Jacques-Joseph Moreau, depicted over 180 men of genius as being diseased. Soon signs of "nervous degeneration" were being discovered among most of the world's leading artists, scientists, writers, and musicians) (Ostwald 1985, 192).

Here we see in Schumann's own self-description the medical model taking over— from madness to mental illness. The precise nature of the illness is endlessly contested, but thereafter, no one questions that it is illness we are talking about.

Knowledge of Schumann's mental state has sharply affected critical reception of his music, especially the music he wrote in the few years before his suicide attempt and incarceration in an asylum, a time when his condition was obviously worsening. Listeners have responded to his music, especially his late music, in four reasonably distinct ways:

Ostwald (1985), clearly the most prolific contributor to this list of diagnoses, also argues that Schumann "had what seems to have been a severely divided self.... Today we would call this a 'narcissistic' or 'borderline' personality disorder" (305).

36. On malaria and tuberculosis, see Neumayr (1995). Syphilis is a common although hotly disputed diagnosis for Schumann. See, among many others, Sams (1971) and Walker (1976).

37. Details of the medical treatments received by Schumann may be found in Ostwald (1985) and Neumayr (1995).

1. The composer is mad and the music is also mad and therefore bad—sick, diseased, deformed, and defective. This corresponds to the traditional notion of disability generally, and madness specifically, as a personal affliction.
2. The composer is mad and the music is also mad and therefore good—visionary, defiant of convention, ahead of its time, divinely inspired. This is the romantic notion of madness as the source and emblem of higher knowledge.
3. The composer is not all that mad, and whatever his psychiatric issues may have been, they have no perceptible impact on the music. This is the prevailing view of current musicology: Schumann's death in a lunatic asylum has unjustly colored the response to his music.
4. The composer's mental differences from the norm are significant enough to place him within a community and tradition of similarly situated artists. His madness is a "dangerous gift."

The first response—that the late music is mad and bad—was prevalent during Schumann's lifetime and has persisted long since. Clara Schumann tried to suppress some of her husband's final compositions out of fear that they were touched by his madness and thus defective. She prevented publication of the Violin Concerto and the Violin Sonata No. 3 and destroyed the Five Romances for Cello.[38] Following Clara Schumann, there has been a long critical tradition that sees in Robert Schumann's music, especially but not exclusively the late music, signs of creative failure and incapacity that mirror his mental state.[39]

A modern variant on this view sees the negative features Schumann's late music as resulting not so much from madness itself as from his attempt to regulate it, to

38. According to Tunbridge (2007, 5),

[Clara's] decision to suppress certain works, such as the Violin Concerto, the Third Violin Sonata and the accompaniments to Bach's Cello Suites, and later to destroy the Five Romances for Cello was taken with the guidance of Joachim and Brahms, and was doubtless driven by a belief that they did not do her husband's talent justice. Certainly Clara's suppression of these pieces has been taken as confirmation that Schumann's creative powers waned, the cause of which invariably is taken to be his mental illness. Schumann's "madness" was never considered to have increased his music's profundity or inventiveness, as was often claimed to be the case with Romantic artists, but to have resulted in a "darkening" of mood and ultimately creative failure.

Likewise, see Ostwald (1985, 261) on Schumann's Violin Concerto:

[Clara] never liked the work, claiming that it had a "defect" and "showed definite traces of [Schumann's] last illness." She even asked Joachim to recompose the work and "make a really magnificent last movement for me," which he refused to do. Eugenie Schumann, the last surviving witness, stated that in the 1880s, when an edition of Schumann's as-yet-unpublished music was under discussion, Clara decreed, "the concerto should never be brought into the open," and said that she wanted the manuscript to be destroyed.

39. Negative responses to Schumann's late music as tainted by his madness are summarized in Jensen (2001, 281–83). In 1865, August Reissmann described Schumann's late music as

channel it artistically. The classicizing tendencies in the late music (in contrast to the Romantic eccentricities of the earlier music) appear as a kind of cover-up, an attempt to resist the madness musically. In Taruskin's (Taruskin 2005, 3:316) words, "'Classicism,' for him, was a retreat from a threatened abyss."[40]

The second sort of critical response—that the music is mad and good—draws on the Romantic association of madness and genius.

> By the beginning of the nineteenth century, madness—for writers, painters, and musicians—was not simply a withdrawal from the distress of everyday life, a protest against intolerable social conditions or against a debilitating philosophy. It had gained a new ideological charge: madness was a source of creative energy. It would be cruel to say that madness had then become fashionable, as it was always the subject of profound anguish, but there is a grain of truth....Madness, for the Romantic artist, was more than the breakdown of rational thought; it was an alternative which promised not only different insights but also a different logic (Rosen 1995, 647).

For many critics, the odd, eccentric, strange elements in Schumann's music—the "wonderful effects of logical incoherence and schizophrenia," in Rosen's words— are among the most attractive and individual features of his music, and have their roots in his incipient insanity.[41] The music, including the music written long before his final breakdown, is mad and good.

"formless and chaotic," traits he attributed to Schumann's illness. Félix Clément argued in 1887 that many of the later works, going back to the Symphony No. 3, "were clearly conceived and created under the influence of his diseased mind." Likewise, see MacMaster (1928), Niecks (1925), and Taylor (1982), all discussed in Jensen (2001).

40. Likewise, see Rosen (1995, 663) with regard to

> ...the problem of Schumann's late revisions of his youthful works. It is understandable that a composer in his forties should have lost sympathy with the work he had written one or two decades earlier. In addition, Schumann's fears of insanity had increased, and the republication of the early works preceded only by a short time his voluntary entrance into a lunatic asylum. In some cases it would seem as if Schumann had gone through the early works to remove anything which might have seemed insane or even odd.

See also Tunbridge (2007, 105):

> As a result, the "classical" forms of his music from the 1850s are diagnosed as dissociative, masking inner turmoil; thematic focus becomes repetition-compulsion; and the reminiscence of melodies is no longer thought a means to achieve coherence but a manifestation of aural hallucination. In a strange reversal of Goethe's famous dictum, Schumann's late orchestral music makes Romanticism healthy, and Classicism sick.

Goethe had famously said, "The classical I call healthy, and the Romantic sickly."

41. In the longer passage from which I have just quoted, Rosen (1995, 648) warns against an autobiographical interpretation of the eccentricities in Schumann's music:

Musicological responses to Schumann's music tend to fall into the third category—the composer may have been mad, but his madness has no perceptible impact on his music. Yehudi Menuhin, who gave the premiere of the Violin Concerto after it was finally published in 1936, assures us that the music is not mad at all, but quite healthy:

> The concerto is a treasure, and I am completely enchanted! It is real Schumann, romantic and fresh and so logically interconnected in every impulse. Thoroughly mentally healthy throughout.... Perhaps one was startled at the time by the audacious harmonies which today's ears do not find at all surprising. I hope there were better reasons than that for putting Schumann into an insane asylum![42]

Likewise, Schumann's most recent American biographer, John Daverio, argues that not only is the late music perfectly normal, that is, typical of Schumann, but that Schumann himself may not have been all that badly off when he wrote it:

> The myth that portrays the late works as a necessary complement to the final illness has been called into question by more recent appraisals of the documentary and musical evidence. According to this view, Schumann's ultimate descent into madness forfeits its status as the last stage in a disintegrating career. If we want to interpret Schumann's life as a drama, the dementia of his last years will function as the *peripeteia* or reversal that occasioned an abrupt interruption in the work that had continued apace until January of 1854. Indeed, anyone who scans Schumann's last diary entries (on the trip to Hanover in late January 1854) for signs of mental decay will be disappointed. Likewise, an unbiased look at the late music will disclose qualities too frequently overlooked: a heightened intensity of expression, a rigorous limitation of thematic materials, and a visionary prefiguration of features associated with later composers including Bruckner, Reger, and even Schoenberg (Daverio 1997, 17).[43]

> Schumann was haunted from the age of seventeen by the fear of going mad. Only at the end of his short life were these fears realized.... In his greatest creative years, from the age of twenty to thirty, he played with the idea of insanity, incorporating elements of madness into his work—his criticism as well as his music—inventing wonderful effects of logical incoherence and schizophrenia. Whatever Schumann's personal disposition, these elements are clearly stylistic rather than autobiographical. We have no warrant for taking them even as superficial reflections of Schumann's private life.

42. Unpublished letter from Yehudi Menuhin, April 18, 1937; original in the City Archives of Bonn. Cited in Ostwald (1985, 261).

43. Likewise, Daverio further observes, "The shifting relationship between Schumann's illness and his working habits should caution us against arriving at hastily drawn conclusions regarding the effects of this illness on the actual substance of his works. Yet it is precisely in the compositions stemming from the second major depressive phase in Schumann's life (1844–46) that many commentators have heard the first signs of a fatal condition.... Not

Daverio contends that Schumann's mental status is irrelevant to the music, that the later music is pretty much the same as the earlier music. But in comparing Schumann's later music to that of Bruckner, Reger, and Schoenberg, Daverio yields a bit to the Romantic notion of the composer as seer, whose mental differences enable a forward-looking late style (see chapter 5 for further discussion).

Although most current Schumann scholarship downplays the connection between Schumann's music and his madness, even casting doubt on the extent of his psychiatric issues prior to his final illness, a countervailing trend from outside of musicology has claimed Schumann as a possessor of a "dangerous gift," that is, one whose mental differences, no longer understood as an illness, are the source of his creative power (Jamison 1996). For these commentators, Schumann's madness does touch his music in significant ways, but more to mark it as distinctive than to stigmatize it. A very recent development is the emergence of a radical critique of psychiatry and the medical model of cognitive, attitudinal, and behavioral difference as "mental illness." Under slogans like "mad pride" and "mental diversity," a condition that would formerly have been medicalized as "bipolar disorder" (one of the many modern psychiatric diagnoses posthumously assigned to Schumann) gets reconceptualized as a "dangerous gift." The impact of this new attitude has yet to be felt to any significant degree in the reception of Schumann's music.

Ravel

In the later years of his life, Ravel experienced a variety of emotional and neurological disturbances that, in an earlier era, would have been understood as forms of madness. Starting around 1927, he began to experience episodes of disorientation and in October 1932 had what was described as a "nervous breakdown" (a diagnosis affirming that the nerves theory of mental and emotional distress was still in force) (O'Shea 1990). Beginning in 1933, his condition worsened and he lost the ability to compose. Not only was his memory impaired, but he also experienced a variety of auditory disturbances, and he consulted the famous French neurologist, Théophile Alajouanine. According to Alajouanine (1948, 232), Ravel was still able to think musically in a sophisticated way, but was unable to express himself musically, in singing, playing, or notation:

> At the peak of his artistic achievement, rich through an abundant and varied work, already classic, which expresses a delicate climate, Maurice Ravel is struck down by an aphasia.... Oral and written language are diffusely impaired, but moderately so, without any noticeable intellectual weakening. Memory, judgment, affectivity, aesthetic taste do

---

even a generally acknowledged masterpiece such as the Second Symphony is exempt from this sort of dubious conflation of life and artwork.... For now it will suffice to say that the presence of works unremittingly optimistic in affect and undeniably masterful in their handling of compositional challenges should, if nothing else, give us pause" (301–302).

not show any impairment to repeated tests. Understanding of language remains much better than oral or written abilities. Writing, especially, is very faulty, mainly due to apraxia. Musical language is still more impaired, but not in a uniform manner. There is chiefly a quite remarkable discrepancy between a loss of musical expression (written or instrumental), and musical thinking, which is comparatively well preserved.

According to Sacks (2007), today neurologists would probably diagnose Ravel as having a form of frontotemporal dementia.[44] Whatever the diagnosis, by the end of his life, Ravel was unable to function musically at all and, indeed, could barely speak.

Contemporary accounts make it clear that Ravel began to experience symptoms of mental disturbance as early as 1927. Here are Ravel's own descriptions, the first in a jocular tone in 1926 and the second entirely serious from 1930:

> Everything is going well here: my housekeeper twisted her foot, one of my Siamese cats (the most vigorous of them), stuffed herself like a pig and came down with gastritis, and the cat's master is on the lookout for cerebral anemia and senility. I send you the most affectionate of my final lucid thoughts (Letter to Roland-Manuel [1936]. Cited in Jourdan-Morhange [1945, 242]. My translation).

> At the rate it was going, the concerto [Piano Concerto in G Major] should have been finished soon. I hadn't counted on the fatigue which suddenly overwhelmed me. Under the threat of dire repercussions: cerebral anemia, neurasthenia, etc., I have been ordered to rest, and above all to sleep.... I will be able to resume work soon, but with greater moderation (Letter to Georges Vriamont, December 5, 1930. Translated and reprinted in Orenstein [1990, 309]).

In the five years that remained until he was no longer able to compose, he wrote a number of major works, including *Boléro* (1928), Piano Concerto for the Left Hand (1929–30), Piano Concerto in G (1929–31), and *Don Quichotte à Dulcinée* (1932–3). In all the vast musicological literature on Ravel, I have seen virtually no attempt to relate alterations in Ravel's increasingly difficult emotional and mental life to his music. The only significant exception of which I am aware is a

---

44. Sacks (2007) writes:

> Maurice Ravel suffered in the last years of his life from a condition that was sometimes called Pick's disease and would probably now be diagnosed as a form of frontotemporal dementia. He developed a semantic aphasia, an inability to deal with representations and symbols, abstract concepts, or categories. His creative mind, though, remained teeming with musical patterns and tunes—patterns and tunes which he could no longer notate or put on paper. Théophile Alajouanine, Ravel's physician, was quick to realize that his illustrious patient had lost musical language but not his musical inventiveness.

programmatic reading by the distinguished pianist, Marguerite Long, of the Concerto for the Left Hand:

> The more one studies this score the more one clearly sees the idea which inspires Ravel and which cancels the disparity between its episodes—the thought of death, the nightmare of fear, and of solitude. He who has followed the slow and cruel dissolution of our friend as I have and seen from afar the distant symptoms which invaded his lucidity will realize, but not without heartbreak, that Ravel has written his destiny into this work. Such a work presupposes perception of the beyond, and as Cocteau has said, "requires acceptance of the ambassadors of the Unknown" (Long 1973, 63).[45]

The contrast to the reception of Schumann's music could hardly be starker. For Schumann, his madness has threatened to engulf critical reception of his late music; for Ravel, the critics have preferred to avert their gaze.[46] Their reticence may be attributed both to the greater stigma associated with intellectual or cognitive disability and to its relative invisibility compared with physical or sensory disability. Ravel criticism thus falls entirely into my third category: the personal experience of disability is walled off as having no impact on the music.

Hikari Oe

If the critics have avoided looking directly at this aspect of Ravel, in the case of Hikari Oe, they have done little but stare. Hikari Oe is the developmentally disabled son of Kenzaburo Oe, a Nobel Prize winning novelist, much of whose fiction has an autobiographical focus on fathers with developmentally disabled sons. Hikari Oe, now in his early forties, is neurologically unusual and would probably be classified as autistic, intellectually disabled, and visually impaired. He has written a series of short pieces in the style of the late eighteenth century that have been

---

45. A similar suggestion has been offered, very tentatively, by Oliver Sacks about *Boléro*:

> One wonders, indeed, whether Ravel was on the cusp of a dementia when he wrote his Boléro, a work characterized by the relentless repetition of a single musical phrase dozens of times, waxing in loudness and orchestration but with no development. Although such repetition was always part of Ravel's style, in his earlier works it formed a more integral part of much larger musical structures, whereas in Boléro, it could be said, there is the reiterative pattern and nothing else
>
> (Sacks 2007, 313–314).

46. Like Ravel, but for a considerably longer period, Aaron Copland was prevented by some form of dementia (probably Alzheimer's disease) from composing during the final years of his life. Also like Ravel, Copland's critics have generally shied away from talking about this phase of Copland's life and especially from speculating on the impact of Copland's incipient dementia on his final works. Copland's late work will be considered in light of his increasingly severe memory loss in chapter 5.

recorded on two CDs, both of which have been bestsellers both in Japan and the United States. Indeed, each was, for a time, the single top selling classical recording in Japan. Oe's story, and particularly the story of his disability, have dominated discussions of his music. Most reviewers have found themselves virtually unable to offer an appraisal, or even a detailed characterization of the music, so overwhelmed were they at the nature of his disability.[47] Most accounts follow the familiar trope of the overcoming of disability cast as inspirational tearjerker: the triumph of the human spirit over adversity. The critical reception of Oe's modest musical achievement is entirely engulfed by the stigmatic trait of his disability.[48]

Tobias Picker

Tobias Picker is a highly regarded and successful contemporary composer, with a distinguished record of operas and instrumental works performed by major ensembles and soloists. His life and career have been shaped in various ways by Tourette's Syndrome, a neurological disorder characterized by physical and vocal tics. Picker has described the stigmatizing effect of his tics on his childhood, and his use of music to cope with and channel them:

> There was this thing that I couldn't control that made me into a freak. In those days, a lot of parents didn't know that the child couldn't control it. They were always telling me to stop it. I couldn't. It made me angry, as though I was disappointing my parents all the time. Nobody knew what it was.... Music saved me. When I played the piano, I didn't have it (Kellow 2005).

Picker's first public discussion of his Tourette's came in Oliver Sacks's book, *Musicophilia* (Sacks 2007). In it, Picker claims Tourette's, not as a personal tragedy, but as a source both of individual identity and creative energy and distinction. According to Sacks (2007, 231):

> Picker feels that his Tourette's enters into his creative imagination, contributing to his music but also being shaped and modulated by it. "I live my life controlled by Tourette's," he said to me, "but I use music to control it. I have harnessed its energy—I play with it, manipulate it, trick it, mimic it, taunt it, explore it, exploit it, in very possible way."

Picker has repeatedly and explicitly claimed Tourette's as part of his personal and musical identity: "the Tourettic elements in my music have grown into something

---

47. See Cameron (1998) for both a summary and an instance of this phenomenon.
48. The concept of "engulfment"—the reduction of a person to his or her disability—is from Garland-Thomson (1997a). See chapter 7 for further discussion.

emotional. I'm now able to harness and control and also build on them" (quoted in Mostel 2005). In response, a small number of critics have tried to find musical analogues for Tourette's in Picker's music.

> Mr. Picker's music resembled that of his teachers [Babbitt, Carter, Wuorinen] in its disjunct lines, atonal harmonies and irregular rhythms. But a barely controlled explosive streak would erupt unexpectedly, piercing the systematic canvas with bursts of intuitive passion. It is tempting to find a parallel in the neurological disorder with which Mr. Picker was born, Tourette's syndrome (Schwarz 1999).

This sort of speculation has been authorized by Sacks, who claims, "If an artist has a condition like this it is very possible it may enter into his art or creativity in some way" (quoted in Schwarz 1999).

For the most part, however, the reception of Picker's music has not been significantly shaped by his disability. But perhaps in the future, critical appraisal of his music might begin to reflect Picker's own attitude toward his disability, not as an obstacle to be overcome, but as a source of creative life and distinctiveness. Such a critical approach, like the stance of the composer, would claim disability as a personal and creative identity.

The composers discussed in this chapter are diverse in their nationality, time period, and musical style. What binds them together is their shared experience of disability and, even more, the shared critical response evoked by their disability. Whether disability has been understood to mar their music or to endow it with transcendent qualities, whether disability is understood to have been overcome or to remain a fundamental source of creative distinctiveness and energy, it has persisted as an inescapable component of critical study. In short, for disabled composers, the disability inflects the critical response, and in consistent, predictable ways.

Beyond the critical response, the music itself has certain shared qualities that emerge from the composers' experience of disability. In many cases, composers express in their music aspects of their experience of their own embodiment: their physical and mental capabilities shape the music they compose. More specifically, composers with disabilities may narrate musically what it is like to live with a nonnormative body. In the following four chapters, I will explore some of the musical stories that composers with disabilities have told.

CHAPTER 2

Musical Narratives of Disability Overcome: Beethoven

DISABILITY AND NARRATIVE

Music has a variety of descriptive powers. It can depict objects and conditions, relate events, evoke moods and bodily states, and tell stories. It can embody and express every aspect of the human condition, including disability. Direct musical representations of disability include the rhythmic pattern known as *alla zoppa* ("in a limping manner"),[1] the high E near the end of the final movement of Smetana's String Quartet No. 1 ("From My Life") that represents the composer's tinnitus (discussed in chapter 1), and Schoenberg's *Todesfall* (experience of death) represented in his String Trio (discussed in chapter 5), as well as the many musical depictions of madness or mental disorder, including melancholy and obsession.[2]

Beyond these vivid, concrete depictions, music has the power to tell stories about disability.[3] One story that music often tells is that of disability overcome: the musical work encounters and triumphs over a potentially disabling musical event. This story involves a dramatic trajectory that moves through disability to a state of

---

1. According to the *New Grove Dictionary of Music and Musicians*, the term *alla zoppa* (from the Italian word for "lame," or "limping") refers to "a rhythm in which the second quaver in a bar of 2/4 time is accentuated." This rhythmic figure is apparently designed to imitate the walk of someone with a halting, asymmetrical gait. *Alla zoppa* is one of the topics named and discussed in Ratner (1980, 85), where it is described as a "short-long, 'limping' figure."

2. Hepokoski (2002, 149) names the first movement of Mozart's String Quartet in D minor, K. 173, and the first movement of Haydn's String Quartet, Op. 20, No. 5 (Hob. III:35), as "instrumental representations of extreme melancholy or even madness." Likewise, the last movement of Beethoven's String Quartet Op. 18, No. 6 is entitled "La Malinconia," and its strange harmonies and sudden mood changes have been widely discussed. For a historical and theoretical discussion of melancholy, see Radden (2002). On musical depictions of obsession, see Howe (2010).

3. In musical scholarship there is a long and contentious history of discussions of music and narrative. For a recent contribution and a summary of previous scholarship, see Almen (2008).

health restored. Narratives of disability overcome begin to appear in music during the first decades of the nineteenth century, most notably in the middle-period works of Beethoven.[4] In this chapter, I will offer close readings of two symphonic movements by Beethoven (from his third and eighth symphonies) and briefer looks at several other works. My aim is to tease out the stories they tell about disability and, in the process, to explore the historical, cultural, and biographical contexts that enable musical narratives of disability overcome.[5]

Before exploring musical narratives of disability overcome, it is worth acknowledging the same narrative at work in literature, particularly novels of the eighteenth and nineteenth centuries. As Lennard Davis has observed, novelistic plots usually involve the restoration of normality after a period of disruption, the reformation of a deformation, that is, the overcoming or cure of a disability:

> Plot functions in the novel, especially during the eighteenth and nineteenth centuries, by temporarily deforming or disabling the fantasy of nation, social class, and gender behaviors that are constructed as norms. The *telos* of plot aims then to return the protagonists to this norm by the end of the novel.... In this sense, the identity of the novel revolves around a simple plot. The situation had been normal, it became abnormal, and by the end of the novel, the normality, or some variant of it, was restored.... The novel as a form relies on cure as a narrative technique.... The process of narrative, then, serves to wound identity—whether individual, bourgeois, national, gendered, racialized, or cultural. Readers read so that they can experience this wound vicariously, so they can imagine the dissolution of the norms under which they are expected to labor.... At the same time, the reader can rejoice in the inevitable return to the comfort of bourgeois norms.... The alterity presented by disability is shocking to the liberal, ableist sensibility, and so narratives involving disability always yearn toward the cure, the neutralizing of the disability (Davis 2003, 542).

Indeed, characters with disabilities are extraordinarily pervasive in literature in general, and in the nineteenth-century novel in particular, including *Jane Eyre* (Bertha and Rochester), *Moby Dick* (Ahab), Frances Burney's *Camilla* (Eugenia), and *The Scarlet Letter* (Chillingworth).[6] Many novels use a secondary character

---

4. Although narratives of cure, recuperation, normalization, and overcoming are especially characteristic of middle-period Beethoven, there are precedents, particularly in the music of Haydn (see Grave [2008] on "recuperation" in a Haydn string quartet). Cure narratives in particular have a long history before Beethoven came onto the scene, stretching back into classical antiquity. For a discussion of cure narratives in medieval literature and music, see Singer (2010). What is new with Beethoven and his contemporaries is the idea of overcoming disability through heroic personal effort.

5. Such narratives are often referred to in the disability literature as "cure narratives." For critical surveys of disability narratives, see Frank (1995), Couser (1997), and Hawkins (1999).

6. A more speculative list of fictional protagonists whom critics have placed on the autism spectrum would include Herman Melville's Bartleby (Garland-Thomson 2004a; Murray 2008), Charlotte Bronte's Jane Eyre (Rodas 2008), Arthur Conan Doyle's Sherlock Holmes (Fitzgerald 2004), and Charles Dickens's Barnaby Rudge (Grove 1987; Murray 2008).

with a physical difference as a foil to a normative protagonist, including Jane Austen's *Persuasion* (the protagonist, Anne Elliot, in relation to her crippled friend, Mrs. Smith), Mary Shelley's *Frankenstein* (the eponymous protagonist in relation to the monster), Charles Dickens's *David Copperfield* (the eponymous hero in relation to Uriah Heep), Robert Louis Stevenson's *Treasure Island* (Jim Hawkins in relation to Long John Silver), and Anthony Trollope's *Barchester Towers* (Arabin in relation to Madeline Neroni).[7] In each of these novels, the narrative trajectory involves a return to a normative state after some abnormality has been normalized: it involves the overcoming of disability.

The sheer number of fictional representations distinguishes disability from other forms of Otherness:

> While other identities such as race, sexuality, and ethnicity have pointed to the dearth of images produced about them in the dominant literature, disability has experienced a plethora of representations in visual and discursive works. Consequently, disabled people's marginalization has occurred in the midst of a perpetual circulation of their images. Curiously, a social erasure has been performed even as a representational repertoire has evolved (Mitchell and Snyder 2000, 6).

Given the extraordinary prevalence of images of disability in the eighteenth- and nineteenth-century novel, and their consistent use as ways of reinforcing notions of normality within a narrative of disability overcome, it will come as no surprise to see similar themes worked out in the music of the same period.

Somewhat more broadly, Mitchell and Snyder have argued that all narrative, irrespective of time and place and artistic medium, may be understood to involve the repair of deviance:

> A narrative issues to resolve or correct a deviance marked as improper to a social context. A simple schematic of narrative structure might run thus: first, a deviance or marked difference is exposed to a reader; second, a narrative consolidates the need for its own existence by calling for an explanation of the deviation's origins and formative consequences; third, the deviance is brought from the periphery of concerns to the center of the story to come; and fourth, the remainder of the story rehabilitates or fixes the deviance in some manner. This fourth step of the repair of deviance may involve an obliteration of the difference through a "cure," the rescue of the despised object from social censure, the extermination of the deviant as a purification of the social body, or the revaluation of an alternative mode of being. Since what we now call disability has been historically narrated as that which characterizes a body as deviant from shared norms of bodily appearance and ability, disability has functioned throughout history as one of the most marked and remarked upon differences that

---

7. On the last of these, see LaCom (1997).

originates the act of storytelling. Narratives turn signs of cultural deviance into textually marked bodies (Mitchell and Snyder 2000, 53–54).

Sandahl and Auslander have made the same point in a particularly pithy way: "The fates of [disabled] characters often include cure, death, or revaluation in the social order, *a metaphorical quelling of the commotion that disability stirs up in narrative*" (Sandahl and Auslander 2005, 4; emphasis added). In what follows, I explore the ways that music, specifically the music of Beethoven, stirs up and quells disability within a musical narrative that closely follows Mitchell and Snyder's four stages: identifying deviance, marking it as problematic, bringing it from the periphery to the center, and repairing it.

DISABILITY AND THE "TONAL PROBLEM"

Disability enters musical narratives in the form of what Arnold Schoenberg called a "tonal problem."[8] The tonal problem is a musical event, often a chromatic note (i.e., a note from outside the principal scale) that threatens to destabilize the prevailing tonality (i.e., the sense of key). Destabilizing tonal problems have been frequently observed in the critical literature and are most commonly associated with the music of Beethoven and Schubert.[9] In each case, the music contrasts its normative content (the notes of the principal scale, behaving in their normal way) with a

---

8. Schoenberg is best known as a modernist composer, perhaps the most influential composer of the twentieth century. In addition, he was an important music theorist, and his ideas about music have been almost as influential as his compositions. He develops the notion of "tonal problem" in Schoenberg (1967, 1946/1984c, 1995).

9. For example, Kerman (1979) discusses what he calls a "sore note" in Beethoven's String Quartet Op. 59, No. 1. More generally, Kamien (2000, 79–80) has observed:

> Beethoven's opening themes frequently generate enormous tension and expectation. Of course, Haydn and Mozart also wrote opening themes that create rhythmic and tonal instability or ambiguity. Yet Beethoven's opening gestures tend to be more extreme in this respect. Beethoven often uses chromatic inflection to build instability, tension or tentativeness directly into opening themes....In the diatonic context of an opening theme these chromatic events are "marked for memory" and are reflected in later themes of the exposition as well as in large-scale tonal motions or key successions.

Kamien adduces as examples a number of works, mostly from Beethoven's middle period, including the two symphonic movements discussed in this chapter. Epstein (1987, 213) makes a similar observation:

> The point of inquiry is whether, in movements that contain chromatic elements as part of their basic pitch shape, this chromatic shape is subsequently reflected in the movement in terms of patterns of modulation and key relationships. Conversely, in movements whose basic shapes do not contain such chromatic elements, are there no, or significantly fewer, such relationships? The evidence strongly suggests a positive conclusion in both cases. In virtually every instance in which Beethoven's initial themes contain a striking chromatic element, this shape is manifested in the large....In contrast, those moments whose thematic shapes are fundamentally diatonic have markedly fewer modulations or key relations that conform to this chromatic pattern.

disruptive, deviant intrusion whose behavior threatens the integrity and normal functioning of the musical body.

For Schoenberg, the tonal problem has two aspects, imbalance and unrest. That these are both bodily states reveals the underlying physicality of Schoenberg's organicist orientation: a piece of music is a human body, and as such is susceptible to nonnormative stigmatized states, that is, disabilities.[10] The normative and desirable bodily state (balance and rest) is understood in relation to a nonnormative and undesirable state (imbalance and unrest).[11]

For Schoenberg, musical works typically begin in a normative state of balance and rest, which is disrupted by the imbalance and unrest of the tonal problem. It is then the task of the piece to solve the problem and reestablish balance and rest.

> Every tone which is added to a beginning tone makes the meaning of that tone doubtful. If, for instance, G follows after C, the ear may not be sure whether this expresses C major or G major, or even F major or E minor; and the addition of other tones may or may not clarify this problem. In this manner there is produced a state of unrest or imbalance which grows throughout most of the piece and is enforced further by similar functions of the rhythm. The method by which balance is restored seems to me the real *idea* of the composition (Schoenberg 1946/1984, 123).

Imbalance and unrest are desirable aesthetically. They propel the piece forward and provide an essential contrast with the normatively balanced and restful beginning and ending. Without a tonal problem to solve, a piece would be lifeless, without character or interest. Just as walking involves a series of controlled falls—without them there would be no forward motion at all—a tonal problem is precisely what enables and impels musical motion. At the same time, however, imbalance and unrest are nonnormative bodily states that require normalization. For the listener approaching the piece from the outside, imbalance and unrest are sources of pleasure and interest, but from the point of view of the piece's tonic, its principal harmony, they are disruptive and potentially disabling events that must be contained, abnormalities abnormalities that must be normalized.

Epstein adduces the *Eroica* Symphony as his principal analytical example, but he discusses many other works as well, all by Beethoven and all from the middle period. With reference to Schubert, Cone (1982) identifies in a short piano piece what he calls a "promissory note," that is, a note "that has been blocked from proceeding to an indicated resolution, and whose thwarted condition is underlined both by rhythmic emphasis and by relative isolation" (236). This particular note, and Schubert's disability-related musical narratives, are discussed in chapter 3.

10. See chapter 6 for further discussion of Schoenberg's metaphorical conflation of a musical work with the human body.

11. It is relevant to note that balance is not only a physical state but also a medical category. During the period between Beethoven's compositions and Schoenberg's theories, a new medical model emerged involving "a new way of seeing the body based on a model of balance in which too much or too little of something caused a disease, while the mean or norm was considered good health" (Davis 2008, 26). See also Canguilhem (1991).

In this sense, Schoenberg's tonal problems are analogous to those secondary characters in literature discussed earlier whose negative qualities, often manifested in physical disabilities of one kind or another, make them useful foils for the normative protagonists. In Shakespeare's *The Tempest*, for example, Prospero says of Caliban, "He is as disproportion'd in his manners / As in his shape" (Act V, Scene 1). Caliban is a narrative problem in much the same way that Schoenberg's unassimilated notes are a tonal problem—he is essential to the forward propulsion of the drama, which would be impoverished by his absence. At the same time, however, Caliban is understood with respect to Prospero and Miranda as a negative figure, and his disability is treated poetically as the stigmatizing outward manifestation of his problematic role in the narrative.

As long as the tonal problem can eventually be solved, with balance and rest restored, the piece emerges enriched, its metaphorical body fully intact. But the aesthetic value of that restoration depends precisely on the threat posed by the tonal problem. If the tonal problem is not understood as at least potentially disabling, then the eventual solution will have little value. For Schoenberg, the eventual triumph over the threat of disability must be won through a struggle:

> The tonic must make great efforts to prevail, just as a revolutionary party after attaining power must make powerless all who at any time had got in its way.... The tonic, once placed in question, must wander through all regions and prevail over every single one after having allowed each to display its full power. And only after conquering and neutralizing all opponents—at the end, in other words—can the power of the tonic prove itself and a *state of rest* again prevail (Schoenberg 1995, 105, 107; emphasis in original).[12]

> The *furtherance of the musical idea* may ensue only if the *unrest—problem*—present in the *Grundgestalt* or in the *motive* is shown in all its *consequences*. These consequences are presented through the *destinies* of the motive or the *Grundgestalt*. Just how the *Grundgestalt* is altered under the influence of the *forces struggling* within it, how this *motion* to which the unrest leads, how the forces again attain a state of *rest*—this is the *realization of the idea*, this is its presentation (Schoenberg 1995, 226; emphases in original).[13]

> Every succession of tones produces unrest, conflict, problems.... Every musical form can be considered as an attempt to treat this unrest either by halting or limiting it, or by solving the problem (Schoenberg 1967, 102).[14]

12. See discussion in Saslaw (1996).
13. See discussion in Saslaw (1997–98). A *Grundgestalt* is a basic musical shape, including melody, harmony, and rhythm. Usually presented at or near the beginning of a composition, it contains the musical ideas that are elaborated and explored in the rest of the music.
14. Likewise, with reference to sonata-allegro form, Schoenberg defines the function of the first theme as that of "formulating the problem of unrest present in the basic gestalt" (Schoenberg 1995, 181).

Over the course of a work, the tonal problem must be solved, and this solution involves normalizing an abnormal bodily state. In that sense, Schoenberg's tonal problem is a concept deeply bound up with disability, both its threat and its actuality. Tonal pieces may thus follow a disability-inflected narrative of bodily balance and rest first asserted, then challenged by imbalance and unrest, and finally restored—a narrative of disability overcome.

MUSICAL NARRATIVES OF DISABILITY OVERCOME

Certain works by Beethoven, especially those of his middle period, grapple with "tonal problems" within a narrative structure that closely tracks Mitchell and Snyder's four phases. The music begins with a relatively straightforward assertion of key. Early on, usually within the first sixteen measures, a chromatic note (i.e., a note from outside the principal, diatonic scale) is stated in a rhetorically charged manner that marks it for attention. In the music that follows immediately, the chromatic note is abandoned, and the music proceeds as if it had never occurred; the normality of the music is apparently unaffected. Later in the work, that chromatic note becomes the focal point for harmonic and formal disruptions that increase in intensity. Finally, near the end of the work, the chromatic note is normalized in some way and subsumed into the diatonic frame.

I want to make three arguments about musical works with this narrative structure. My first argument is historical: musical narratives in which a tonal problem is overcome can be understood in relation to concurrent developments in the history of disability in Europe in the early decades of the nineteenth century. As discussed in the Introduction, historians of disability have identified the early nineteenth century as a time of a paradigm shift in the social and cultural construction of disability. Prior to that period, disability had been construed as something monstrous and unnatural, a permanent and immutable mark of divine disfavor. Beginning in that period, disability was understood as something abnormal, a deviation from the statistically predominant. As such, disability came to be seen as not necessarily permanent; rather, it could be ameliorated—the abnormal body could be normalized.

The history of disability is thus the primary site for the emergence of the concepts of normal and abnormal, concepts that are both embodied in and encouraged by developments in the arts, including music. The musical narrative of disability overcome can be understood as a reflection of, and artistic construction of, the concepts of normal and abnormal. Specifically, the works by Beethoven discussed in this chapter give expression to the possibility, one that was new around the beginning of the nineteenth century, that disability could be overcome or, in musical terms, that the tonally abnormal could be normalized.

The dramatic plan of these pieces can be related not only to the overarching concepts of normal and abnormal but to specific contemporary cultural trends in the conceptualization and treatment of people with disabilities, including the emergence of disability as a concept, the growing awareness of people with disabilities as defining a distinctive class, and the emergence of medical and educational institutions for people with disabilities. These new institutions are based on the belief, one that was new at the time, that through personal effort, and with institutional support, a person with a disability can participate in normal society. In other words, the late eighteenth and early nineteenth centuries mark the first historical era in which disability is understood as *something that can be overcome*. That new understanding is crucial for the narrative structure of the Beethoven pieces to be discussed here, in which the potentially disabling chromaticism is typically overcome through the agency of a vigorous diatonic reassertion.

My second argument is biographical. A dramatic plan that involves the attempted recuperation of disability can be productively understood in part as a musical response to the composer's own disability. This approach is encouraged by Beethoven himself who, in an oft-quoted remark from an 1806 sketchbook, wrote, "Just as you are plunging yourself into the whirlwind of society, and even as it is now possible for you, despite all social obstacles, to compose operas—let your deafness no longer be a secret—even in art" (quoted and discussed in Jander 2000). The literature on Beethoven has long recognized some sort of link between the changes in Beethoven's life (i.e., his deafness) and changes in his musical style. His middle period, often called his "heroic" period, begins with his realization that his hearing loss is serious and permanent, and critics have suggested that the heroism of his musical style reflects his personal heroism in the face of increasingly difficult life circumstances. As Solomon (1998, 162) claims, "[Beethoven's] deafness was the painful chrysalis within which his 'heroic' style came to maturity." Despite this general supposition about Beethoven's musical style, however, few critics have attempted to interpret individual works as expressive of Beethoven's personal experience of deafness.[15]

My third argument involves reception: pieces with this dramatic plan have often elicited critical responses that engage metaphors of disability. From the beginning, listeners have understood the initial chromatic intrusion as something akin to a threat to the bodily integrity of the music, a threat that the remaining music is obliged to resist and, if possible, overcome.

In what follows, I offer brief critical interpretations of several works by Beethoven from the first decades of the nineteenth century. These works share a balanced,

15. A notable recent exception is Jander (2000, 29), who argues that in the third movement of Fifth Symphony "Beethoven uses his music most intensively to confront his experience of going deaf." Jander argues that the remarkable passage that leads from the end of the third movement to the great C-major blast of triumph at the beginning of the fourth gives musical expression to the three symptoms of deafness of which Beethoven had complained: buzzing and rumbling in his ears, expressed in a strange, recurring figure in the violins and violas; difficulty in hearing soft sounds, expressed in the unusually protracted low dynamic level; special difficulty in hearing high-pitched sounds, expressed in the gradual vanishing of upper registers. According to Jander, the sudden brightening into radiant, heroic C-major at the beginning of the fourth movement represents "Beethoven's ritualized triumph over deafness" (43).

diatonic beginning, the intrusion of a tonal problem leading to extensive harmonic disruptions and formal "deformations," and a restorative denouement in which the tonal problem is solved, the wound is healed, the disability cured, the balance reestablished, the rest restored, and the abnormal normalized.[16]

BEETHOVEN, SYMPHONY NO. 3 IN E-FLAT MAJOR, OP. 55 ("EROICA"), FIRST MOVEMENT

The first movement of Beethoven's Symphony No. 3 enacts the narrative of disability overcome in heroic mode: the tonal problem is solved in triumph. Most narrative accounts of the work (and there are a remarkable number) imagine it as depicting a battle or a struggle of some kind.[17] The opening chords and the noble theme that follows are widely understood to introduce us to the heroic protagonist of a drama (possibly Hector, Napoleon, or Prometheus).[18] The music is thus metaphorically conflated with the body of a human being.

The deviant C-sharp that enters in the seventh measure of the piece (the fifth measure of the heroic theme) is the first chromatic note in the piece and has become the locus for intensive interpretive activity. Some commentators liken the C-sharp, and the indecisive harmony it supports, to the hero's external surroundings, possibly a cloud (Tovey) or a fog (Oulibicheff).[19] Of greater interest in the present context, many commentators imagine the C-sharp as expressive of something that more directly inflects the hero's journey, something that causes him to pause or hesitate. The hero strides forth, but then falters momentarily, his mobility impaired either by an external obstacle or an internal apprehension or foreboding.[20]

> The [hero-idea] steps forward in the violoncellos still pale, not yet warming, like the rising sun level on the horizon—as though hiding itself in chilly haze. This "not yet"

16. The term "deformation," to refer to anomalies in musical form, is taken from Hepokoski and Darcy (2006). See chapter 6 for discussion.

17. The relevant literature is surveyed and evaluated in Sipe (1992, 1998) and Burnham (1995). See also Hyer (1995), Earp (1993), and Lockwood (1982).

18. The identification of the narrative hero as Hector is a conceit of Arnold Schering (1933). The narrative hero has been identified as Napoleon by many commentators, including A. B. Marx (1859/1979). Schleuning (1987) and Floros (1978) have argued that the narrative hero is the mythical Prometheus, conflated with the historical Napoleon.

19. "Then, as the violins enter with a palpitating high note, the harmony becomes clouded, soon however to resolve in sunshine. Whatever you may enjoy or miss in the *Eroica* Symphony, remember this cloud" (Tovey 1935, 30). "After presenting itself, like the sun on the horizon, it holds itself for a moment behind the fog of an indecisive harmony" (Oulibicheff 1857, 175, quoted and translated in Sipe 1998, 61–62).

20. In their summaries of the relevant critical traditions, Sipe (1998) associates the C-sharp with a sense of apprehension before battle and Burnham (1995) associates it with an intimation of eventual death.

(how often Napoleon spoke it in the heat of battle, if his generals called for the reserves too early!), this dispersal in the relative minor of the dominant, expands the phrase from four measures to thirteen; we are directed toward great situations (Marx 1859/1979, cited and translated in Sipe 1992, 257).

Simple and upright [the motive] goes forward; from its first step it is marked with the seal of its destiny, that marches to its appointed end and knows no other. The soul into which this order has entered bends, at the fifth bar, under the burden. But this burden itself is its destiny, is a part of its essence; it accepts it with a sigh, and abandons itself to the stream (Rolland 1929/1956, 55, cited in Sipe 1992, 257).

In the local context, the hero regains his balance and continues to stride forth. Later, however, that C-sharp engenders a series of harmonic and formal disruptions that represent the vicissitudes of the hero's journey. In the end, the C-sharp and its implicit threat to the hero's mobility are overcome in a blaze of triumph and affirmation.

Who is this hero, and what is the impediment that causes him to hesitate, the burden under which he bends? Some critics have identified Beethoven himself as the hero and his deafness as the obstacle to be overcome. Shortly before he wrote this symphony, Beethoven underwent a spiritual crisis brought about by his growing deafness. In a remarkable personal statement known as the *Heiligenstadt Testament* (named for the small town near Vienna where it was written), Beethoven lamented his fate, contemplated suicide, but decided to continue living for the sake of his art. Critics have imagined the *Eroica* Symphony as a musical reenactment of this document:

The *Heiligenstadt Testament* is a leave-taking—which is to say, a fresh start. Beethoven here metaphorically enacted his own death in order that he might live again. He recreated himself in a new guise, self-sufficient and heroic. In a sense, [the testament] is the literary prototype of the *Eroica* Symphony, a portrait of the artist as hero, stricken by deafness, withdrawn from mankind, conquering his impulses to suicide, struggling against fate, hoping to find "but one day of pure joy" (Solomon 1998, 157–58).[21]

Solomon's interpretation of the *Eroica* Symphony as a portrait of the composer struggling to overcome his own fate, specifically his incipient deafness, forms part of an interpretive tradition that is epitomized by an earlier, French critic, Romain Rolland.[22] For Rolland, Beethoven himself is the protagonist of the drama ("In a mind like that of Beethoven, wholly absorbed in itself, its passions, its combats, and its God, the external world counts merely as a reflection, an echo, a symbol of the interior drama") and the *Eroica* emerges directly from the *Heiligenstadt Testament* as

21. The tradition of interpreting the *Eroica* Symphony in relation to the *Heiligenstadt Testament* extends back to J. W. N. Sullivan and beyond: "The *Eroica* Symphony is an amazingly realized and coordinated expression of the spiritual experiences that underlay that document" (Sullivan 1927, 134–35).

22. For a compelling account of Rolland's position within the interpretive traditions around the *Eroica* Symphony, see Sipe (1992, 236):

an expression of Beethoven's determination to overcome the effects of his deafness ("In the lone house at Heiligenstadt, a death-roar is wrung from Beethoven. A mournful Testament... The appealing cry of the Testament is answered by the mysterious horn-call of the *Eroica*") (Rolland 1929/1956, 53, 38).

For Rolland, the hesitation and wavering of the C-sharp in measure 7 are directly associated with Beethoven's deafness, and the ensuing musical response with Beethoven's determination to overcome it.

> Hesitation of the still troubled soul to follow the injunction given it by the invisible Master, the call to action, to the great destiny!... And this throws the light of day on the "October night" [Roland refers to Beethoven's authorship of the *Heiligenstadt Testament* in October of 1802] in which the bleeding heart of Beethoven received, in a clap of thunder, the heroic mission, and, for a moment, grew faint and wavered.... But the imperious flood takes possession of him again and carries him along (Rolland 1929/1956, 40).

Rolland's language may now seem a bit overblown, but I think his basic insight is sound: the first movement of Beethoven's *Eroica* symphony traverses a narrative of disability overcome.

For Solomon, Rolland, and the others, Beethoven's crisis, in both its prose and musical expression, is entirely personal: deafness is his private tragedy, his effort to overcome it his personal victory. But Beethoven is operating in a larger social and cultural context, in which the ongoing reconceptualization of disability plays a major part. In 1802, the idea that a disability can be overcome, that an abnormality can be remediated and thus functionally normalized, was something new in the history of disability and in the history of ideas. In Beethoven's lifetime, in all of the European capitals, new institutions for the education and training particularly of the blind and the deaf were springing up, embodying the possibility of remediation and recuperation. Vienna itself was home to a newly created *Taubstumminstitut*

The psychological approach was heightened to the pitch of eloquence by Romain Rolland. Rolland accepted Wagner's abstract, metaphorical program from 1851. But he argued that Wagner's allegorical hero was in fact Beethoven himself. The psychological background for the work became for Rolland Beethoven's struggle with his deafness and his victory through art. Rolland used the *Heiligenstadt Testament* as evidence that Beethoven "fought" his fated affliction to a "heroic" victory with the composition of the Third Symphony.

A similar link between the *Testament* and the *Eroica*, and the resulting narrative of personal striving in the latter, is described in Downs (1970, 603): "The dramatic purpose of the *Eroica* Symphony is to provide a lesson on the conquering of self... The forces which so nearly overwhelmed Beethoven, and which ultimately resulted in the *Heiligenstadt Testament* and the rejection of suicide as a way out of difficulty, certainly appear in the musical parable."

designed to assist "deaf-mutes" in overcoming their condition by providing them with the skills necessary to make them functional members of the larger community.[23] Beethoven's *Heiligenstadt Testament* and his *Eroica* Symphony can both be understood in part as emblems of this new way of thinking about disability.

This new way of thinking is evident in Beethoven's life as in his music, as he sought a variety of technologies (i.e., adaptive prostheses) to overcome his disability.[24] This effort was also part of a general contemporary trend toward the use of technology as a means of remediating and rehabilitating people with a variety of disabilities. Stiker (2000) describes a variety of such "normalization devices" for different disabilities, and situates them within the larger history of the rehabilitation of disability:

> The idea of remedial training or rehabilitation for the disabled was then not new, but it put down solid roots, for some categories at least, at the end of the Age of Enlightenment.... Through the intervention of appropriate techniques, people with sensory disability could gain access to an intellectual, artistic, professional life.... The examples of the blind and the deaf put us on a route toward the twentieth century, with the themes of rehabilitation and specialized institutions. But training, especially in the form of conventional schooling, which was a principal goal of these foundations, was still very far from what we, today, would call reintegration and redeployment. Then it was a matter of drawing impaired persons out of inactivity and lack of culture, the results of prejudice concerning their capacity. The implications are more humanist and moral than social. The disabled are to be "raised up," restored.... Even on the level of praxis, a change was in the offing [by the end of the eighteenth century]. A sharper scientific focus, the more effective medical treatment of many afflictions, *the will no longer to accept as destiny what is made in society and can be modified by it*—all this favored what we might call a humanization of the lot of the aberrant, a willingness to address these situations through appropriate technology (Stiker 2000, 104–108; emphasis added).

This new attitude toward disability, including deafness, one that refuses "to accept as destiny what is made in society," can be heard in the triumphant response of the *Eroica* Symphony to its initial, troubling C-sharp. In this way, Beethoven is understood to thematize his own deafness within his music, and he does so in accordance with this new way of thinking about disability. The *Eroica*'s narrative of disability overcome thus forms part of the history of disability, and that history in turn provides an essential context for the interpretation of Beethoven's life and work.

23. For a contemporary account of the *Taubstumminstitut,* see Pezzl (1923, 274–77). Among their therapeutic activities, the residents of the *Taubstumminstitut* operated a printing press that printed opera libretti, among other things. For more on institutions for the deaf in general, see Branson and Miller (2002) and Lane (1984).

24. For a recent account of Beethoven's deafness as it changed over time and his attempts to remediate it using contemporary technology, see Ealy (1994).

BEETHOVEN, SYMPHONY NO. 8 IN F MAJOR, OP. 93, FINALE

The final movement of Beethoven's Symphony No. 8 enacts the same drama of disability overcome, but in a comic mode. As in the *Eroica* Symphony, critical reception of the Finale of the Eighth Symphony has often invoked narratives of human actions and human bodies, including bodies that are disabled or threatened with disability, and a rhetorically charged C-sharp sets those narratives in motion in both pieces. That the same C-sharp is the tonal problem in both works suggests a kinship between them. Indeed, in its treatment of disability, the Eighth Symphony Finale can be heard as a humorous, ironic deflation of the heroism of the *Eroica*.

In the Eighth Symphony's Finale, C-sharp bursts forth in measure 17 as a shocking surprise—a *fortissimo* outburst amid a quiet diatonic surrounding—and is not resolved, or musically acknowledged in any way, in its local context. It is clearly felt as an interpolation (the music would move smoothly if it were simply excised) and critics have generally understood it as a manifestation of brusque humor. Tovey (1935, 66) calls the C-sharp a "stumbling block," thus foregrounding the idea of loss of physical balance and the possibility of a fall. Instead of the threat of tragedy implicit in the *Eroica*'s C-sharp, this C-sharp suggest something more like a spill, a tumble, a pratfall (as Scott Burnham has called it).

Rosen (1980, 337) describes it as "an irritant," a description that Burnham (2001b, 135) qualifies this way:

> I prefer to hear the initial C-sharp less as a portentous irritant and more as a musical pratfall. The suddenness both of its onset and its disappearance renders the C-sharp more a potentially comic interjection than a real threat (compare, for example, the equally famous D-sharps at the outset of the Violin Concerto), although one could make a case for the reactive vehemence of the statement of the theme that immediately follows. Perhaps a conflation of both views comes out about right: brutal humor.

Burnham goes on to imagine the C-sharp as evoking some of the crude humor traditionally associated with people who are hard of hearing: "a nearly deaf man reacting with pique to a conversation that has fallen out of his range of hearing: 'What?!' " (Burnham 2001b, 135). In light of Beethoven's own deafness, there is obviously considerable irony here, as Burnham acknowledges. The C-sharp may be taken as an emblem of deafness, of Beethoven's own deafness (just like the C-sharp in the *Eroica* Symphony), but rather than a potential tragedy to be heroically overcome, it is rendered here as a source of crude humor.

The intrusive C-sharp leads eventually to the tonicization of F-sharp minor in the coda, and an astonishing expansion of the form. As Rosen (1988, 342) puts it: "When we consider the violence of this climax [in F-sharp minor], we no longer may judge the length of the coda as unprovoked; we may see it as justified and even demanded by the material. From bar 17 on, the grandest of all Beethoven's codas is a necessity." In other words, the initial "tonal problem" leads both to harmonic abnormalities and to formal "deformations."[25]

For Tovey, as for Rosen, the deformation and the humor of the greatly enlarged coda have their source in the "abnormal" C-sharp of measure 17:

> With all its originality and wealth, there has so far been no puzzling or abnormal feature in the movement, with one glaring exception. What on earth did that irrelevant roaring C-sharp mean? Thereby hangs a tail, videlicet, a coda that is nearly as long as the whole body of the movement. My pun is not more violent than Beethoven's harmonic or enharmonic jokes on this point (Tovey 1935, 67).

In his description of the F-sharp minor culmination of the coda, and its extended normalization within the overall tonic, Tovey emphasizes the comic effect. In particular, he imagines an outburst of laughter among the gods as they see the lame Hephaestus walking about.

> The main theme reaches that C-sharp; and now it suddenly appears that Beethoven has held that note in reserve, wherewith to batter at the door of some immensely distant key. Out bursts the theme, then, in F-sharp minor. Can we ever find a way home again? Well, E-sharp (or F natural) is the leading note of this new key, and upon E-sharp the trumpets pounce, and hammer away at it until they have thoroughly convinced the orchestra that they mean it for the tonic. When this is settled, in sails the radiant second subject again. Now Ganymede is all very well; but the original cup-bearer of the gods is Hephaestus, who is lame, and grimy with his metallurgy in the bowels of the earth. However, he will not be ousted; and so the basses sing the theme too. Straightway unquenchable laughter arises among the blessed gods as they look at him bestirring himself about the house. The laughter has all the vaults of heaven wherein to disperse itself, and to gather again into the last long series of joyous shouts (Tovey 1935, 67).[26]

Thus, Tovey and Burnham agree that disability is the source of humor in this work, either a hearing impairment (Burnham) or a mobility impairment (Tovey). As in the *Eroica*, a narrative involving disability is set in motion by a "tonal problem," specifically a C-sharp that can be associated either with a mobility impairment or deafness. But the shared narrative is inflected very differently in the two sym-

---

25. As noted earlier, the term "deformation" comes from Hepokoski and Darcy (2006), and will be discussed in chapter 6. For a fascinating study of the Beethovenian coda as a "narrative prosthesis," that is, a compensatory response to a marked deviance, see Quaglia (2007). The concept of narrative prosthesis originates with Mitchell and Snyder (2000). See also Wills (1995).

26. For a study of Hephaestus in relation to classical and more recent attitudes toward disability, including its potential for farce and low humor, see Ebenstein (2006). Like deafness, mobility impairment is often played for laughs in literature.

phonies. Indeed, one can imagine the last movement of the Eighth Symphony as an ironic inversion of the first movement of the Third Symphony: what was once treated as potential tragedy now returns as something akin to farce, and the abnormal is normalized amid "unquenchable laughter."

In artistic representations, people with disabilities are generally forced to conform to a small number of familiar stereotypes, which Sandahl and Auslander (2005) call "cultural scripts." One of the most widely circulated of these scripts is the Heroic Overcomer—the person with a disability is the protagonist of an inspirational tale of the triumph of the human spirit over adversity. If we were to imagine the *Eroica* Symphony as a person with a disability, this is the cultural stereotype it would be understood to enact (although, as we have seen, in 1802 this role was new, not yet a stereotype). Another familiar script involves the role of what Norden (1996, 20) calls the Comic Misadventurer: "a disabled person victimized by one or more able-bodied people, and a disabled person whose impairment leads to trouble, whether self-directed, other-directed, or both. All in the name of comedy, of course." There is a long tradition, in literature and film, of treating certain disabilities, including hearing impairments, as a source of comedy. In this sense, were we to imagine the Finale of Beethoven's Symphony No. 8 as a person with a disability, it would be a Comic Misadventurer.

SOME OTHER WORKS

Beethoven used a similar narrative of disability overcome in a variety of works, mostly from his middle "heroic" period, after he had become aware of his progressive loss of hearing. An interesting earlier work, from 1795, is one of the piano trios from Beethoven's first published work, his Opus 1. The second movement of the second of these trios begins in a bright-toned, relaxed, pastoral mode (the key is E major). The first hint of trouble comes in the fourth measure, with three gentle iterations of B-sharp, a note from outside the main scale and used here as a subtle intensification of C-sharp, a note from inside the scale. The embellishing function of the B-sharp is clear, and it resolves normally, but it is rhetorically charged by virtue of its three-fold repetition—this insistence frames it as a tonal problem.

Shortly after, this tonal problem bursts out in a way that threatens to explode the pastoral calm by disrupting the musical form in the most profound way. This movement (like the others discussed in this chapter) is cast in one of the standard and standardized forms of the period, known now as "sonata form." This form is constrained by certain conventions governing the relations among the keys. The first half of a sonata-form movement in a major key is expected to end five steps higher than it began (in this movement, which begins in E major, the first half should end in B major). The second half is expected to end in the home key (in this case, back in E major). The tonal problem posed by the B-sharp threatens to overturn both of these conventions in a highly destabilizing way.

Toward the end of the first half of the movement, we have arrived safely in the expected B major. Then, the problematic B-sharp, respelled as C-natural, pushes the music toward the unexpected and remote key of G major, where the first half ends.[27] Toward the end of the second half, at a moment when the piece is supposed to be confirming its home key, C-natural asserts itself in a particularly shocking, violent way to become the tonic note of a new, unexpected key. The second formal half thus threatens to end not in the home key of E major but in the profoundly problematic key of C major. In response to this disruption, Beethoven adds a supplementary section to the form, a coda, which undertakes strenuous, repeated efforts to regain the tonic, E major. At the very end, in the last few measures, an expressive turn toward E minor brings in a C-natural. C is the last chromatic note in the movement, as B-sharp was the first, and only in the final four measures is it normalized within the framework of the home key, E major.

Looking at the narrative in dramatic terms, we hear a chromatic note insinuate itself early in the work. It has no immediately apparent consequences, but later bursts forth in increasingly violent and destabilizing ways, threatening the integrity of the form. Ultimately, the piece does succeed in normalizing its abnormal elements, but only with considerable effort, and with a sense of lingering cost. The narrative is still one of disability overcome—much of the tonal energy of the work is directed toward precisely that end—but there is no sense of triumph. The disabling tonal problem proves virtually intractable. The piece never fully recovers from its deformities, never fully solves its tonal problem—it remains a disabled body until the end, and the work ends in tragedy rather than triumph. This work might be said to be about disability, but not about Beethoven's own deafness, which was not yet manifest. And the notion that disability might be triumphantly overcome is not yet part of the mix.

In many other works, Beethoven confronts tonal problems (symbolically representing disabilities) in a variety of ways and with a variety of outcomes. His Violin Concerto is in D major, and the D-sharps that enter in measures 10 and 12 of the first movement are marked for attention in various ways. D-sharp is the first chromatic note in the movement, and it enters following a sweet, simple, lyrical, rhythmically normal, diatonic scalar passage. It is the first note played by strings, and played in a markedly unidiomatic way—in imitation of the timpani. As Dubiel

27. "A nonresolving exposition," according to Hepokoski and Darcy (2006). For Hepokoski and Darcy, this movement exemplifies an "S-deformation"—S stands for Second Theme:

> These involve cases in which S begins normatively, in the proper "new key," then "loses" that new key *permanently* by wandering away from it and/or shifting elsewhere.... In all cases the subsequent recapitulation is deeply problematized....S starts out in the normative B major (measure 26) but this key is subjected to slippage and crisis. No B PAC [perfect authentic cadence in B-major] occurs, and the exposition ends with a PAC in the "wrong key" G major (!) (measure 39). These problems produce an even more dire nonresolving recapitulation later in the piece—one of the earliest in the repertory (Hepokoski and Darcy 2006, 142).

(1999) observes, the D-sharp is hard to interpret harmonically, so divorced is it from the tonally normal music before and after. It is not even clear if the note is functionally an E-flat (as in Beethoven's original notation) or a D-sharp (as in the published score).

And once heard, the D-sharp is almost immediately forgotten, with no obvious consequences—the music resumes its smooth, diatonic course as though nothing had happened. "This degree of registral, timbral, rhythmic, and motivic synthesis makes it hard to know whether the pitch D-sharp remains an issue. How can it not be, sounding as odd as it does? Yet the music makes no mention of D-sharp for an amazingly long time after this cadence [in measure 18]" (Dubiel 1999, 266).

The D-sharp does have consequences later, but not by creating the sort of intense instability familiar from other works with similar tonal problems. Rather, the Violin Concerto's D-sharp is normalized fairly early in the narrative, and is provided a logical harmonic explanation within D-major. Here is Tovey's (1949b, 384) description: "The mysterious unaccompanied D sharp near the beginning of the Violin Concerto is unharmonized, and flagrantly avoids explanation until a later harmonized passage explains it as an example of sweet reasonableness."

There is a striking disparity in this work between the intensity of the tonal problem—those mysterious timpani-like D-sharps in measures 10 and 12—and the relatively subdued response. The principal consequence is the tonicization of E-flat in the development section, a formal section that normally contains remote modulations in any case. The E-flat is quickly normalized within the tonic-affirming return of the opening music, and the D-sharp/E-flat irritant is hardly heard from again.

In the Piano Concerto No. 5 in E-flat major, a tonal problem posed by the chromatically lowered sixth degree of the scale, C-flat, is repeatedly introduced, elaborated, and normalized. The C-flat is introduced (in the local context of E-flat minor) fairly early in the orchestral introduction to the first movement, and it leads to a series of modulations to C-flat as the tonic of a new key, spelled either as B major or B minor. The most potent of these modulations involves the entire second movement, which is in B major. Throughout all three movements of the work, Beethoven is concerned with a contrast between the normal sixth degree of the scale (C) and the chromatically altered version of the same degree (C-flat). This duality has a powerful symbolic charge, as William Rothstein observes: "I have the strong sense that C-natural is intended as the 'healthy,' extroverted version of the neighbor note; C-flat, if not exactly 'sick,' is at least inward-looking and incapable of decisive action" (personal communication).

Early in the first movement of Beethoven's Trio Op. 70 ("Ghost"), an unexpected, chromatic, problematic F-natural intrudes into a bright, brilliant, bravura D major. The intrusion is rhetorically marked by a sudden change of texture to a single sustained note, a radical cessation of activity that highlights the F. The harmonic meaning of the F is initially unclear, and efforts to define it (i.e., to rationalize and normalize it) become the focus of the musical narrative.

In its local context, the music continues back in diatonically unimpaired D major, although now in a lyrical rather than a heroic mode. Later, however, the tonally problematic F creates significant harmonic disruptions, most notably a tonicization of the F itself as the culminating event of the development section. Within the recapitulation, a greatly expanded transition to the second theme is the context for the rectification and recuperation of the tonal problem posed by the intrusive F. This work thus follows the familiar narrative path of disability overcome (following Mitchell and Snyder): identifying deviance, marking it as problematic, bringing it from the periphery to the center, and repairing it.

In all of the works discussed in this chapter, the narrative of disability overcome unfolds within the conventional outline of the sonata form. This form emerges from a desire to create and resolve musical tension on the largest scale. The essential imperative of the form is that music heard in a nontonic key in the first part of the form must be heard again in the tonic in the last part of the form. The normalization of the tonal problem thus coincides with this larger formal thrust toward normalization.

As noted earlier, there is a potent analogy to the literary form of the novel, which emerged at the same time as the sonata form, in response to similar social forces, and with similar cultural impact:

> If we accept that novels are a social practice that arose as part of the project of middle-class hegemony, then we can see that the plot and character development of novels tend to pull toward the normative. For example, most characters in nineteenth-century novels are somewhat ordinary people who are put in abnormal circumstances, as opposed to the heroic characters who represent the ideal in earlier forms such as the epic.... The novel form, that proliferator of ideology, is intricately connected with concepts of the norm. From the typicality of the central character, to the normalizing devices of plot to bring deviant characters back into the normal of society, to the normalizing coda of endings, the nineteenth- and twentieth-century novel promulgates and disburses notions of normalcy and by extension makes of physical differences ideological differences (Davis 1995, 42 and 49).

The cultural work of the novel is, in part, to assert the normality of its central characters in distinction to abnormal Others. The sonata form, in its central dialogue between normal procedures and "deformities" does the same kind of work: it normalizes the abnormal. Sonata form simultaneously reflects these concepts and assists in constructing them. As Beethoven employs the form in the works discussed here, the sonata form, with its inherent thrust toward normalization, becomes the medium through which tonal problems—those potentially disabling events—may be heroically overcome in triumph, or treated as a subject for high or low comedy, or allowed to create musical disruptions that are scarcely recuperable.

CHAPTER 3

Musical Narratives of Disability Accommodated: Schubert

A "PROMISSORY NOTE" IN A *MOMENT MUSICAL*

In Schubert's *Moment Musical* in A-flat major, D. 780, No. 6, the failure of the E-natural in measure 12 to resolve to F as expected, although hardly noticed in its local context, initiates a series of increasingly disruptive harmonic moves. The most extreme of these moves is a modulation to E major, where the tonally problematic E, distant from the original key of A-flat major, becomes the tonic of a remote new key. The end of the piece contains a return to A-flat major, but it is insecurely reattained—the resonance of the deviant E-natural is felt right to the end of the work and beyond.

In a widely read essay, Edward Cone identifies the E-natural as what he calls a "promissory note," that is, a note "that has been blocked from proceeding to an indicated resolution, and whose thwarted condition is underlined both by rhythmic emphasis and by relative isolation" (Cone 1982, 236). In Cone's interpretation, this work

> dramatizes the injection of a strange, unsettling element into an otherwise peaceful situation. At first ignored or suppressed, that element persistently returns. It not only makes itself at home but even takes over the direction of events in order to reveal unsuspected possibilities. When the normal state of affairs eventually returns, the originally foreign element seems to have been completely assimilated. But that appearance is deceptive. The element has not been tamed; it bursts out with even greater force, revealing itself as basically inimical to its surroundings, which it proceeds to demolish (Cone 1982, 239–40).

Cone relates this dramatic plan to "the effect of vice on a sensitive personality," and, specifically, to Schubert's experience of syphilis, including its disabling psychological and physical effects.

A vice, as I see it, begins as a novel and fascinating suggestion, not necessarily dangerous though often disturbing. It becomes dangerous, however, as its increasing attractiveness encourages investigation and experimentation, leading to possible obsession and eventual addiction. If one now apparently recovers self-control, believing that the vice has been mastered, it is often too late: either the habit returns to exert its domination in some fearful form, or the effects of the early indulgence have left their indelible and painful marks on the personality—and frequently, of course, on the body as well (Cone 1982, 240).

The term "vice" is apparently Cone's subtle reference to Schubert's sexual promiscuity—whether gay or straight is a matter of current debate.[1] Schubert's "vice," in this reading, proves impossible to repress, and bursts forth with destructive consequences, including the indelible and painful bodily markers of syphilis. The progress of Schubert's bodily experience of illness and the progress of his music follow the same path, of an encounter with and response to disability.

Cone's promissory notes are a particular kind of "tonal problem," a rhetorically charged chromaticism that engenders harmonic and formal disruptions. Cone does not offer a simple one-to-one mapping of the tonal problem onto a particular disability, or even to the psychological anxiety that may be induced by the threat of disability. Rather, he understands the tonal problem as setting in motion a narrative that can be usefully interpreted in terms of disability, including the composer's own personal experience of disability.

Schubert's narratives of disability, however, are somewhat different from those of Beethoven, discussed in the previous chapter. For Beethoven, disability is to be struggled with and, if possible, overcome, and his works often take on the personality of the Heroic Overcomer. For Schubert, given his different experience of disability and his different musical inclinations, disability is not something that can be unequivocally overcome. Rather, it is something that must be lived with, accommodated. Its traces can never be expunged, but leave a permanent mark on the musical body, just as syphilis marks the physical body. As a result, when Schubert grapples musically with disability, his works are more likely to enact the cultural script of the Saintly Sage (Norden 1996), in which disability confers a supranormal wisdom. In Schubert's music, there is a sense that wisdom is something otherworldly, to be won only through suffering.

PIANO SONATA IN B-FLAT MAJOR, D. 960

The first movement of Schubert's Piano Sonata in B-flat major famously engages with G-flat as a disruptive tonal problem. The disquieting trill on G-flat in

1. The current conversation about Schubert's sexuality begins with Solomon (1989). Solomon's argument, and Schubert's sexuality, remain controversial topics. See, for example, McClary 1993.

measure 8 and its generative implications have been widely discussed.[2] In Rosen's words:

> The opening phrase of the first theme of this movement ends with a trill in the bass, *pianissimo*, on a G-flat resolved into an F, and the more one plays it, the more the entire work seems to arise out of that mysterious sonority. The long passage in F-sharp minor [at the beginning of the second theme area] works out the implications of the opening theme on the largest scale (Rosen 1980, 249).

These implications, both formal and harmonic, include both the apparent second theme in F-sharp minor, alluded to by Rosen, and a protracted episode in D minor near the end of the development section.

Even as the narrative of Schubert's music involves normalizing the tonally problematic G-flat and the unusual harmonies to which it gives rise, critical response to this music has often involved attempts to normalize them analytically.[3] The musical narrative itself and the long tradition in Schubert studies of attempting to rationalize Schubert's harmony in relation to prevailing (usually Beethovenian) norms involves both Schubert and some of his critics in the emerging history of the concept of the normal. The relationship of G-flat (and its associated harmonic areas) to the sonata's tonality, like the relationship of Schubert's characteristic harmonies to tonality in general, has been understood as abnormal, requiring musical or analytical recuperation. Thus, the expressive impact of the work depends on understanding the G-flat as a serious breach in the integrity of the musical body.

After exploring (or perhaps indulging in) unusual harmonies and keys to which the G-flat gives rise, the music of the first movement makes an effort to heal that breach. Specifically, at the end of the movement, the music makes a number of attempts to create a convincing final cadence in B-flat major, each of which

---

2. Among recent discussions, see Webster (1978–79), Rosen (1980), Kerman (1986), Fisk (2001), and Kopp (2002). Neff (2001, 287–88) offers a Schoenbergian analysis that emphasizes the capacity of the G-flat to "endanger the power of the tonic."

3. Cohn (1999) includes a brief survey of critical responses to Schubert's harmony generally and to the harmonic consequences of the problematic G-flat in the Piano Sonata in B-flat major specifically. These responses fall roughly into three categories, all of which recognize the challenge posed by Schubert's music to normative (Beethovenian) tonal harmony: 1) attempts to reconcile Schubert's harmonies with tonal norms; 2) celebrations (or condemnations) of Schubert's harmonies for their independence from tonal norms; 3) creation of alternative, nontonal theoretical frameworks. Cohn's article represents the third category. For an example of the first category, in which Schubert's harmony is analytically normalized (i.e., understood in relationship to classical norms), see Fisk (2001, 19):

> Because of Schubert's manifest characterological differentiation of keys other than tonic and dominant from those fundamental keys, and because in his mature music he still accords to tonic and dominant their traditional structural roles, he does not simply relegate classical tonal and formal procedures to a peripheral, frame-producing status. Instead he explores his own idiosyncratic tonal paths and creates space for these explorations against the persisting and palpable background of the tonic-dominant axis.

dissipates in silence. Finally, the music provides two strong perfect authentic cadences, both featuring a normatively resolving G-flat. The disruptive potential of the G-flat would seem to be fully contained at this point—now it is presented as a simple chromatic upper neighbor—and its abnormality would appear to be fully normalized.

But the movement continues with a three-fold reminiscence of the opening theme. As the third of these concludes, the ominous trill on G-flat returns, in virtually every respect just as it was in the beginning. The tonal problem has not been solved—its imbalance and unrest resound right through the end of the movement. Certainly there is no sense at all of heroic overcoming in the Beethovenian manner. If the G-flat can be understood metaphorically as a wound of some kind, as I shall argue, then the wound remains open, unhealed at the end of the movement. The musical body remains in a nonnormative, stigmatized state—it is still disabled. But the disability, instead of being cured in triumph or mourned as a personal tragedy, is accepted and accommodated.

The tonal problem posed by the G-flat resonates throughout the entire multi-movement work. In the Finale, the tonal problem is revisited for the last time. In Alfred Brendel's description,

> In the touching epilogue [measures 490–511], which seems to suspend time before the final *stretta*, the three-note descent [G–G-flat–F] emerges as a serious question. The ensuing bars subtly make us aware that G-flat has ceased to pose a problem, and the sonata's "*Dolens*" (as I would call it) is finally overcome (Brendel 1990, 75–76).

But despite Brendel's reference to a problem "overcome," the Finale's treatment of the G-flat seems more an almost light-hearted reminiscence, an attempt to laugh off a problem that was treated in all seriousness in the first movement. In this sense, the Finale stands in somewhat the same relationship to the first movement that Beethoven's Eighth Symphony's Finale does to the *Eroica's* first movement—a humorous and ironic commentary on what had previously seemed a potential or real tragedy.

PIANO TRIO IN B-FLAT MAJOR, OP. 99 (D. 898)

The less-discussed Piano Trio in B-flat Major, Op. 99 (D. 898), is a virtual companion piece to the Sonata, both in terms of structure and narrative. Both works date from the end of Schubert's short life, when his syphilis, and the arduous contemporary treatments for it, were taking a heavy toll. The first movement of the Trio begins in heroic mode, but soon bumps up against an ominous, trilled G-flat (measure 9). As in the Sonata, the G-flat engenders a variety of harmonic and formal deviations.

In sonata form, one of the most significant moments comes at the beginning of the final large section. This is a culminating point in the formal drama, the beginning of the recapitulation, when the opening music returns in the principal key. Usually coming after a period of harmonic wandering and emotional intensification (the development), the recapitulation usually comes as a moment of clarification and release, predicated on a double return: the original tune comes back in its original key.

In the Piano Trio, this double return is dramatically overturned. As the development section ends, the music stands on F; this is the dominant note of the main key, B-flat, and is the note most likely to lead back to B-flat, just where we expect the music to go. That F is embellished with its chromatic upper neighbor, G-flat, recalling the tonal problem of the opening, but treating the G-flat in a normative way, as a decoration of the structurally superior F. Then, as the recapitulation approaches, the relationship between the F and G-flat is surprisingly reversed: the G-flat ceases to decorate F and, instead, the F leads to G-flat. Just as that reversal starts to sink in, the opening music enters, signaling the beginning of the recapitulation. But, astonishingly, it enters in the wrong key! The tonally problematic G-flat has apparently managed to hijack the form, diverting the music from the normative B-flat to a new, remote key of which the G-flat itself is the unlikely tonic. It would be hard to imagine a more significant "sonata deformation."[4] As in the Sonata, the situation is eventually rectified, but the problematic G-flat continues to leave traces until virtually the end of the movement.

In both the Sonata and the Piano Trio, there is no Beethovenian sense of vindication through struggle. Rather, the narrative has been inflected to suggest resigned accommodation rather than heroic triumph. A rhetorically marked G-flat ruptures and destabilizes a previously secure, diatonic B-flat major. This tonal problem then leads to a variety of harmonic dislocations and formal deformations. In the end, however, the tonal problem is not overcome, but accepted and accommodated.

METAPHORS OF DISABILITY

These musical differences—Beethoven's sense of overcoming as opposed to Schubert's sense of accommodation—are reflected in the metaphors critics have used to understand these works. In the two Beethoven symphonies discussed in chapter 2, critics have understood the tonally problematic C-sharp as a form of blockage, an obstacle in a heroic progress toward a goal. In the Schubert sonata, in contrast, critics have understood the problematic G-flat as a puncture or opening in a metaphorical container, and the container operates in two relevant senses. First,

4. The term, as noted earlier, is from Hepokoski and Darcy (2006). The relationship between F and G-flat in the Trio is discussed extensively in Sly (2001). Sly interprets the thematic return in G-flat at measure 187 as still part of the development section, and contends that the structural recapitulation does not begin until the tonic returns in measure 211. But even in this view, the separation of the thematic and harmonic returns in itself comprises a "sonata deformation."

the protagonist is freed or banished from a confining or protective enclosure and forced to wander. Second, the puncture permits toxic foreign elements to enter the bodily enclosure from outside.

Many theories of tonal music imagine a key to be a kind of container, in the same way that a body can be understood as a kind of container: things are either inside or outside the container, and are separated by a boundary.[5] If a key is a container, then it contains the seven diatonic notes and the harmonic progressions they can form, with such progressions bounded by a cadence (Saslaw 1996). In that sense, chromatic "promissory" notes and "tonal problems" are intrusions from outside the container. They rupture the protective external boundary of the tonic key just as a sharp object pierces skin.

That sense of a boundary transgressed, a container suddenly opened, is felt consistently in critical descriptions of the G-flat trill and its aftereffects. For Fisk, for example,

> Schubert finds a context for his mysterious gesture that makes its G-flat not merely a coloristic element, but a seemingly portentous one. The trill—Schubert's particular trill, so low, so hushed, so close to stopping time—reconfigures a common chromatic inflection, the lowered sixth degree, as something extraordinary. The G-flat emerges beneath the first semicadence as a harbinger of *something outside or beyond* what is implied by the theme itself, something fascinating in both its allure and its danger (Fisk 2001, 241–42; emphasis added).

Inside the diatonic container of the first theme is peace and security, outside is danger, and it is the trilled G-flat that opens the container.

Metaphorically, the puncture of a container is a wound. By rupturing the diatonicity of the tonic key, tonally problematic notes like Schubert's G-flat threaten the integrity of the musical body, and create an opening that permits the contents of the container to leak out or, perhaps, permits an outside infection to enter. Although this is not a direction that Schubert criticism has taken in the past, I would suggest that, in this sense, tonal problems may provoke an anxiety about bodily integrity comparable to and closely related to the anxiety provoked by the contemplation of wounds or disabilities in one's own—or in another's—body. Contemplating these chromatic notes, in all of their challenging deviance from the prevailing diatonic norm, is like contemplating deviance of any kind and may produce the kind of terror associated with bodily dissolution. These intrusive chromatic notes may

---

5. As Mark Johnson (1987, 21) observes, "Our encounter with containment and boundedness is one of the most pervasive features of our bodily experience. We are intimately aware of our bodies as three-dimensional containers into which we put certain things (food, water, air) and out of which other things emerge (food and water wastes, air, blood, etc.)." See chapter 6 for a discussion Johnson's brand of philosophical "experientialism" and its implications for both music and disability.

cause us to think about our own bodies, about the wounds and disabilities to which they are subject.

The G-flats of the Sonata in B-flat major and its companion Piano Trio in B-flat major convey very much the kind of musical meaning that Cone attributes to his "promissory" E-natural in the *Moment Musical* No. 6. In all three works, the narrative may be understood in relation to Schubert's syphilis, the disabling disease that impaired his health in many different ways and eventually killed him.

> It is well established that Schubert suffered from syphilis. The disease was probably contracted late in 1822, and although it was ameliorated by treatment, or perhaps just by time, it was, of course, in those days, incurable. Did Schubert's realization of that fact, and of its implications, induce, or at least intensify, the sense of desolation, even dread, that penetrates much of his music from then on? (Cone 1982, 241).[6]

Even more specifically, I want to hear in the G-flat itself one of the "indelible and painful marks on the personality—and frequently, of course, on the body" left by this disease (Cone 1982, 240). Syphilis manifests itself in many ways and, in Schubert's case, left many marks on his body at different times, including a genital chancre within a month of the initial infection, a rash of pinkish, circular spots roughly a month later, followed by further eruptions of inflamed, dome-shaped papules on various parts of his body, including his face and head, leading eventually to hair loss.[7] All of these external marks would have been recognized by both physicians and laypersons as symptoms of syphilis, and Schubert himself doubtless understood them as the stigmatizing outer marks of a disease that was virtually certain to destroy his health and to cause his premature death. In Schubert's poignant words,

> I feel myself the most unhappy and wretched creature in the world. Imagine a man whose health will never be right again, and who in sheer despair over this ever makes things worse and worse, instead of better; imagine a man, I say, whose most brilliant

6. Likewise, see Gibbs (2000, 93, 109):

> While it is impossible to offer definitive posthumous diagnoses, especially in a case where compromising materials may have been intentionally destroyed, physicians and biographers, after examining the surviving evidence, have concluded almost unanimously that Schubert contracted syphilis, possibly in late 1822. The various specific references to his symptoms and treatments—rashes, aches and pains, and so forth—are consistent with the primary and secondary stages of the disease.... Even if the medical treatments Schubert received, probably including applications of a highly poisonous mercury salve, were helpful, his view of the world was nevertheless altered, and he apparently believed that his time was limited. As tests to verify the healing of venereal diseases were not yet available, one can reasonably speculate that Schubert consciously embarked on his final creative stage, a period customarily associated with the autumnal glow of later years, when he was only in his mid-twenties.

7. There is a significant secondary literature on Schubert's health issues, including his syphilis. See Hayden (2003), Bevan (1998), and Sams (1980).

hopes have perished, to whom the happiness of love and friendship have nothing to offer but pain, at best, whose enthusiasm (at least of the stimulating kind) for all things beautiful threatens to disappear, and I ask you, is he not a miserable, unhappy being?[8]

Schubert would also have shared the common understanding that syphilis is contracted through sexual contact, which introduced "alien substances" or "poisons" into the body and blood (Sams 1980, 17).[9] Through the metaphor of the container, the B-flat major key of the sonata can be understood as analogous to a body, possibly Schubert's own body. The tonally problematic G-flat can therefore be heard as a puncture in the container, a wound in the metaphorical body. "Alien substances" and "poisons" may enter through the wound and seriously compromise the normal functioning of the musical body, which must reacts as best it can to heal itself. Ultimately, however, there is no cure, no heroic overcoming, just acceptance and accommodation.

Following Cone's lead, I have argued for hearing in the sonata and the trio a narrative of a bodily experience of disease and disability. A much more prevalent metaphorical hearing of Schubert's music identifies him as a Romantic Wanderer and hears in his music a recurring tale of "exploration, banishment, exile, and eventual homecoming" (Fisk 2001, 267).[10] This literature emphasizes Schubert's feeling, lived in his life and expressed in his music, of being an outcast, isolated from the community, in a state of exile, always and forever an outsider.

What is the source of this sense of alienation, loneliness, and inalterable otherness? What impels the wanderer on his journey? An important strain in recent Schubert scholarship has suggested that the answers to these questions may be found in his culturally stigmatized and legally forbidden homosexuality (Solomon 1989). I would like to suggest that the same feelings are also among the most widely shared and discussed responses to personal experience of disability (including disabling diseases, such as syphilis).[11] Certainly, it is well established that Schubert's physical withdrawal from society at various points during the 1820s was directly

8. Letter to Leopold Kupelwieser on the last day of March 1824, after Schubert had been seriously ill for more than a year. Cited in Sams (1980, 17), where it is adduced as a response to "the secondary stage of the disease [which] would now be extending and tightening its grip."

9. Sams cites contemporary medical treatises on syphilis, including those written by Schubert's own doctors, Josef von Vering and Ernst Rinna. Likewise, Bevans (1998) describes bleeding, purging, and emesis (along with mercury) as the principal contemporary treatments for syphilis, all ineffective against the disease and harmful to the patient. According to Bevans, "The main objective of all the measures used was to rid the body of the toxins or poisons produced by the disease" (250). To put it in the metaphorical terms of my own discussion, something undesirable from outside the bodily container had entered through an opening; the cure depended on expelling the foreign element, moving it from inside to outside.

10. See also Kinderman (1997).

11. Stiker (2000, 8) observes, "Disability strikes me in that very elementary and perhaps unsophisticated need not to be exiled, misunderstood, strange and a stranger, in my own eyes at first, then in the eyes of others." Certainly Beethoven experienced and spoke of his deafness as isolating: "I was soon obliged to seclude myself and live in solitude.... I must live quite

related to his desire to hide the stigmatizing marks of his disease (Sams 1980). Indeed, the profound experiences of alienation, banishment, loneliness, wandering, isolation, and unalterable otherness would seem to be something that gay culture and disability culture share in common. Whatever role Schubert's sexuality may have had in shaping the narrative trajectory of his music, and whatever the nature of that sexuality, his experience of disability also played a formative role.

---

alone and may creep into society only as often as sheer necessity demands; I must live like an outcast" (*Heiligenstadt Testament*, October 1802). Likewise, "In my present condition I must withdraw from everything" (letter to Karl Amenda, July 1801) and "I am living—alone—alone—alone! Alone! Alone!" (letter to Karl August Varnhagen von Ense, July 1812). All cited and discussed in Solomon (2003, 61). In this sense, both Beethoven and Schubert find themselves inhabiting a realm apart, what Sontag (1978, 3) refers to as the "kingdom of the sick": "Illness is the night-side of life, a more onerous citizenship. Everyone who is born holds dual citizenship in the kingdom of the well and in the kingdom of the sick. Although we all prefer to use only the good passport, sooner or later each of us is obliged, at least for a spell, to identify ourselves as citizens of that other place."

CHAPTER 4

Musical Narratives of Balance Lost and Regained: Schoenberg and Webern

INVERSIONAL SYMMETRY AND BALANCE

In the traditional, tonal music of the nineteenth century, the musical narrative often hinges on key: the music departs from and returns to a principal key, and that journey may take many different forms. As we have seen, the departure may be motivated by a tonal problem and the return may be associated with an effort to overcome that problem. Toward the beginning of the twentieth century, a new kind of music—atonal music—began to emerge. This is music that is relatively unconcerned with key and has no particular tonality. Such music is often concerned instead with the relations among its motives or themes. At a deeper level, atonal music often engages a sense of what is known as "inversional symmetry."

Imagine all the pitches arranged vertically from the lowest to the highest. If one of those pitches were established as a midpoint, we could imagine the other pitches arranged symmetrically around it. For example, if the D that lies in the middle of the piano keyboard (also the second lowest string on the violin) were established as a central pitch, we could imagine that the F-sharp four semitones above it would be balanced by the B-flat four semitones below it, that the A seven semitones above it would be balanced by the G seven semitones below it; in short, every pitch would have a partner equidistant on the opposite side of the D. In such a situation, looking upward from D would appear the same as looking downward from D: that is inversional symmetry.

In a large body of atonal music, inversional symmetry comes to function in a manner analogous to key in tonal music: a systematic way of regulating the relationships among the tones, a normative principle of pitch organization.[1] And, as with any normative principle, inversional symmetry may be subject to deviation and disruption.

---

1. Inversional symmetry as an organizing principle in post-tonal music has been widely theorized, most extensively by George Perle and David Lewin. Perle observes that inversional symmetry

The atonal music of Schoenberg and Webern, written between 1908 and the outbreak of World War I, often narrates the establishment, disruption, and reestablishment of a normative symmetry. This narrative may be present only in part; pieces may unfold without any significant disruption of symmetry, or their symmetry may be disrupted and never reestablished, or a sense of symmetry may gradually emerge without ever having been clearly established in the first place. The initial sense of balance may be precarious, the disruption not vividly marked, the structural response not notably violent, and the resolution not entirely definitive.

In all of these situations, the interplay between a normative symmetry and abnormal disruptions can be usefully understood in relation to the cultural construction of disability. In all of the literature on musical symmetry, there is an emphasis on balance, on the physical sense of symmetrical balance around a fulcrum, of a body in a physically balanced state. In this context, deviations from inversional symmetry are felt as physical disruptions that unbalance the musical body, and create the threat (or the reality) of a disability. Inversional symmetry and symmetrical balance thus create the possibility for musical narratives that depend on a contrast of normative and nonnormative bodily states. Atonal music is typically understood as pure abstraction, devoid of cultural or social meaning. Through its reliance on inversional symmetry, however, this music both reflects and participates in the cultural and social construction of disability.[2] In what follows, I will explore narratives of balance lost and regained in three atonal works by Schoenberg and Webern.

WEBERN, BAGATELLE, OP. 9, NO. 5

Webern's Bagatelle, Op. 9, No. 5 (1911–13) begins in a state of perfect pitch symmetry around D.[3] Indeed, the notes of the piece, for the first four measures, simply

---

...can serve as the foundational premise of a coherent and natural twelve-tone harmonic language, just as the triad does for the harmonic language of diatonic tonality; and just as the universality of the triad presents diatonic tonal music with a normative principle that defines the meaning of dissonance—a controlled departure from the triad, which remains the referential norm even when it is momentarily absent—so can analogous departures from symmetrical relations provide a basis for prolongational procedures in twelve-tone tonal music (Perle 1996, xiv).

Perle is referring to his own brand of "twelve-tone tonality," but his remarks about the normative force of inversional symmetry have wide application in post-tonal music. See also Perle (1991). Lewin's approach to the topic will be discussed in chapter 6.

2. Scherzinger (1997) makes a similar argument about the role of inversional symmetry in dissolving traditional gender binaries embodied in the major-minor duality of traditional tonality, and relates pitch inversion to a contemporary interest in sexual inversion.

3. The initial symmetry in this piece has been noted by Antokoletz (1984), Morgan (1992), Stoecker (2003), and Davies (2007).

move outward in opposite directions from that central tone, thus vividly establishing a normative sense of inversional balance: C-sharp is balanced against D-sharp, C against E, B against F, and B-flat against G-flat. The balance is disrupted in measure 5 by the viola's C, ten semitones above the center. This is the highest and (although marked *pianissimo*) the loudest note in the piece so far. It thus takes on a special rhetorical charge and sense of urgency. In order to maintain the sense of balance around D, that C must find its inversional partner E, and preferably the E that lies ten semitones below the center—that is the note needed to maintain the pitch symmetry. Until then, the music gives a sense of being off balance, its initial symmetry impaired.

The sense of symmetry around D waxes and wanes over the course of the piece and several potential arrivals on E present themselves. The desired E, ten semitones below the center, does arrive at the very end of the piece, but the final chord contradicts rather than confirms the original D-symmetry. The narrative of the piece is thus one of balance established, disrupted, and only partially and equivocally restored; the abnormal is never fully normalized.

WEBERN, MOVEMENTS FOR STRING QUARTET, OP. 5, NO. 2

The second of Webern's Movements for String Quartet, Op. 5 (1909) begins in a similar state of inversional symmetry and balance. The axis of symmetry is again D, with every note balanced by its inversional partner: G with A, B with F, and A-flat and D with themselves. The arrival of C-sharp signals a forceful disruption of the symmetry. Rhetorically marked as a melodic highpoint under a fermata, the C-sharp has no inversional partner, thus creating a musical gesture of passionate seeking: the C-sharp seeks to balance itself with an E-flat.[4]

The music that follows arrives on several different E-flats, but none is fully satisfactory. At the end of the piece, however, the C-sharp itself returns, and within a fully symmetrical structure. The final chord, with C-sharp once again under a fermata, is arranged symmetrically in pitch: A balances E and the low C balances the fermata C-sharp. C-sharp is now fully and satisfactorily balanced by C, although it was never successfully balanced by E-flat, despite repeated attempts. The basic narrative structure of balance established, disrupted, and then restored still shapes the piece, but with a twist: the balance that is enforced at the end is not exactly the same as the one that was disrupted at the beginning. In this music, the forces of normal

---

4. Lewin (1982–83) is the source for much of this discussion, including the idea that the C-sharp seeks an appropriate E-flat to maintain the inversional balance established in the opening. See also Archibald (1972), who describes the power of symmetry in this piece to create a situation in which "we expect near-symmetries to become completed" (159) and in which "we expect completion of symmetrical groupings when there seems to be an imbalance" (160).

and abnormal, balance and imbalance, symmetry and asymmetry, ability and disability, are evenly matched.

SCHOENBERG, "VALSE DE CHOPIN," FROM *PIERROT LUNAIRE*

The opening of the "Valse de Chopin" from Schoenberg's *Pierrot Lunaire* (1912) projects a strong sense of symmetry around A. In the first four beats of the piece, we hear eight different notes, and these are arranged symmetrically around A, with one significant exception: the D-sharp that lies eighteen semitones above the center has no inversional partner to balance it. The desired pitch would be another D-sharp, eighteen semitones below the center and thus thirty-six semitones (i.e., three octaves) below the original, unpartnered D-sharp.

In the music that immediately follows, both the sense of symmetry around A and of D-sharp as a rhetorically charged challenge to it are intensified. The aggregate of all twelve tones is heard repeatedly in this piece, which also moves rapidly to fill out the entire pitch space from its lowest to its highest note. As the music moves toward its close, there are two fleeting iterations of the long-sought D-sharp (measures 32–33), and then, as the first line of text returns, the missing D-sharp is stated prominently on the downbeats of three successive measures. The arrival is not entirely conclusive, but nonetheless it suggests the tentative culmination of a narrative arc set in motion by the initial challenge to inversional symmetry.

The issues of symmetry and balance, of bodily integrity and disability, posed by the music of "Valse de Chopin" resonate also with its text, explicitly concerned as it is with disease. The text likens a diseased body to a disturbing piece of music. The first line of the text, with its disruptive "drop of [tubercular] blood on the sick man's lip" ("Wie ein blasser Tropfen Bluts/Färbt die Lippen einer Kranken") is thus associated musically with the disruption of inversional balance and the ambiguous attempt of the music to restore it.

SYMMETRY AND BALANCE IN THE THEORETICAL TRADITIONS

Like Schoenberg and Webern's free atonal music itself, the theoretical traditions that have grown up around it have also been preoccupied with inversional symmetry and balance. Those traditions may be said to begin with Schoenberg himself. For Schoenberg, a tonic in a tonal piece and an inversional axis in an atonal piece are both capable of inducing a musical sense of harmonious balance, and in analogous ways. As Lewin (1968, 2–3) observes:

> The "balance" of the total chromatic induced by the functioning of such an inversion was treated by Schoenberg, throughout his career, as something quite analogous to the

balance induced by a tonal center.... [Schoenberg] conceived of a "tonic" as a fulcrum about which all else balanced.... Indeed, the widely used term "tonal *center*" implicitly suggests exactly such a notion.[5]

In many musical situations, tones can be understood as balanced on a central fulcrum.

For Schoenberg, operating within the organicist tradition, a piece of music is analogous to a human body, and as such is susceptible to nonnormative stigmatized states such as imbalance. The normative and desirable bodily state (balance) is understood in relation to a nonnormative and undesirable state (imbalance). And although imbalance may be understood as desirable in many contexts, permitting the forward motion both of human bodies and musical works, if excessive and uncontained, if incapable of normalization, imbalance may become disabling.

Schoenberg believed that musical works typically begin in a normative state of balance, which is disrupted by what he called a "tonal problem" (as discussed in chapter 2). Schoenberg is generally concerned with *tonal* problems, that is, with threats to tonality, and his descriptions generally assume the presence of a major or minor key. Nonetheless, the concept (including Schoenberg's own description of it) can be extended to the disruptions of an atonal symmetry as well: "Every succession of tones produces unrest, conflict, problems.... Every musical form can be considered as an attempt to treat this unrest either by halting or limiting it, or by solving the problem" (Schoenberg 1967, 102). Over the course of "every musical form," the tonal problem must be solved, and this solution involves normalizing an abnormal bodily state: rest is reattained and balance is restored.

From this point of view, the atonal works by Webern and Schoenberg discussed here can be understood as musical bodies with potentially disabling "problems." The C in Webern's Bagatelle, the C-sharp in Webern's Movement for String Quartet, and the D-sharp in Schoenberg's "Valse de Chopin" are all rhetorically charged notes that challenge and disrupt a prevailing inversional symmetry. In terms of narrative, they are problems to be solved, abnormal elements to be normalized, and disabilities to be remediated or rehabilitated. In each case, however, the musical response to the problem is ambiguous.

5. Lewin relates the idea of inversion to other tonal theorists who invoke the concept of balance, including Jean-Philippe Rameau (for whom dominant and subdominant are balanced symmetrically around a tonic) and Hugo Riemann (whose harmonic dualism imagined a major and minor triad generated symmetrically above and below a root). The role of inversional symmetry in dualist theories of tonal harmony and in early theories of atonal music is explored in Bernstein (1993). Lewin's own theoretical work, centrally concerned with inversional balance and thus implicitly engaging the normative and nonnormative body, will be discussed more fully in chapter 6.

In traditional tonal music, particularly the music of Beethoven, tonal problems are often solved in a triumphant blaze, as discussed in chapter 2. Schoenberg and Webern, however, have a different way of dealing with problematic disruptions of the normative scheme. Their music offers narrative engagement with issues of disability, but without the promise that the disability can be overcome, much less in a heroic manner. An initial symmetry, once lost, proves difficult or impossible to reattain. The music may express a concomitant sense of regret and loss, and the affective context is more one of melancholy recollection than bitterness or anger. Schoenberg and Webern's free atonal music, so often resistant to straightforward narratives of overcoming, is expressive of a more open, accepting attitude toward disability. The music creates an artistic space within which disability can be accommodated.

THE GROTESQUE AND THE DEGENERATE

The subtle narratives of disability embedded in the free atonal music of Schoenberg and Webern intersect in complex and interesting ways with two other related cultural categories: the *grotesque* and the *degenerate,* which are themselves intertwined.[6] A surprising number of early modernist musical works, including Schoenberg's *Pierrot Lunaire,* reveal a pervasive preoccupation with common grotesque features, including disease, deformity, and disability (see, for example, the separate settings by Franz Schreker and Alexander von Zemlinsky of Oscar Wilde's *Birthday of the Infanta,* with its central figure of a hunchbacked dwarf). This tendency is even more pronounced in the visual arts of the same period, where an interest in the grotesque, including the deformation and distortion of the human form, is a defining characteristic. As art historian Frances Connelly (2003, 2, 6) observes,

> Images gathered under the grotesque rubric include those that combine unlike things in order to challenge established realities or construct new ones; those that deform or decompose things; and those that are metamorphic....Grotesque describes the

6. For a history of the concept of the grotesque and its role in twentieth-century opera, see Fullerton (2005). Draughon (2003) describes the waltz, the ostensible genre of Schoenberg's "Valse de Chopin," as a locus for the grotesque and the degenerate, and further describes the close linkage between degeneracy and disability on the one hand and femaleness and Jewishness on the other:

> At the turn of the century, this rural-urban polarity was intimately bound with ideologies of gender, the body, and decadence. While the *Stadtmensch's* body came to be regarded as a potential carrier of a feminized, urban degeneracy, the ideology of *Korperkultur* (body culture) proposed a cure for this degeneracy in an idealized chaste and rural male body (Draughon 2003, 390).

On the role of the waltz in Schoenberg's music as "a parody of its former self" and as "signifying *horror*," see Cherlin (1998, 593).

aberration from ideal form or from accepted convention, to create the misshapen, ugly, exaggerated, or even formless. This type runs the gamut from the deliberate exaggerations of caricature, to the unintended aberrations, accidents, and failures of the everyday world represented in realist imagery, to the dissolution of bodies, forms, and categories.... The grotesque permeates modern imagery, acting as punctum to the ideals of enlightened progress and universality and to the hubris of modernist dreams of transcendence over the living world.[7]

The paintings of Oskar Kokoschka and Richard Gerstl, for example, both close associates of Schoenberg's, frequently involve distortions of the human form that invoke the tradition of the grotesque. In this, they exemplify a pronounced trend in artistic Expressionism toward extreme emotional and bodily states.

The artistic tradition of the grotesque frequently involves depictions of people with disabilities. According to Lennard Davis (1997b, 64),

> One of the ways that visual images of the disabled have been appropriated into the modernist and postmodernist aesthetic is through the concept of the "grotesque."...While the term *grotesque* has had a history of being associated with [a] counterhegemonic notion of people's aesthetics and the inherent power of the masses, what the term has failed to liberate is the notion of actual bodies as grotesque. There is a thin line between the grotesque and the disabled.

Schoenberg's own paintings, particularly the well-known series called "Gazes," involve severe deformities and distortions of the human face and thus engage the grotesque directly. One of the most persistent distortions involves unbalancing the symmetry of the two eyes. In the frequently reproduced "Green Self-Portrait" (1910), for example, much of the face is dematerialized in favor of a vivid representation of the eyes, and these are strikingly asymmetrical. These asymmetrical depictions of the human form are related to the musical asymmetries discussed above: in both cases the body (physical or musical) is thrown off balance, and some of the resulting artistic energy resides in the tension between a normative state of symmetrical balance and the challenge to normativity posed by asymmetry and imbalance.[8]

7. For additional discussions of the grotesque in the visual arts and music, see Powell (1974), Schorske (1981), and Sheinberg (2000).
8. In an important recent book, published after the foregoing was written, Siebers (2010) argues that art is identifiably modern precisely and fundamentally because it represents and finds beauty in the nonnormative, fractured, disfigured, disabled human body:

> My argument here conceives of the disabled body and mind as playing significant roles in the evolution of modern aesthetics, theorizing disability as a unique resource discovered by modern art and then embraced by it as one of its defining concepts. Disability aesthetics refuses to recognize the representation of the healthy body—and its definition of harmony, integrity, and beauty—as the sole determination of the aesthetic. Rather, disability aesthetics

Asymmetry, whether in music or in painting, would have been understood by Schoenberg and his contemporaries as an outward mark of *degeneracy,* a politically charged, pseudoscientific term typically used to condemn aspects of modern life and art (Pick 1989). Here is part of a description by Max Nordau, from his widely circulated treatise on *Degeneration* (1892), of the physical symptoms and disabling abnormalities associated with degeneracy:

> Degeneracy betrays itself among men in certain physical characteristics, which are denominated "stigmata," or brandmarks.... Such stigmata consist of deformities, multiple and stunted growths in the first line of asymmetry, the unequal development of the two halves of the face and cranium.... In the mental development of degenerates, we meet with the same irregularity that we have observed in their physical growth. The asymmetry of face and cranium finds, as it were, its counterpart in their mental faculties. Some of the latter are completely stunted, others morbidly exaggerated (Nordau 1892/1993, 16–18).

Asymmetry, as a deviation from a normative state of symmetry, a deformation of a form, is where the cultural traditions of the grotesque and the degenerate intersect most forcefully with disability. Far from rejecting bodily asymmetries and the degeneracy they were understood to suggest, Schoenberg and Webern's music embraces them. In its acceptance of musical asymmetry and its willingness to forego the narrative restoration of a normative symmetry, this music accepts and accommodates the kinds of bodily differences that were culturally marked as grotesque or degenerate.

TWELVE-TONE MUSIC, INVERSIONAL SYMMETRY, AND DISABILITY

Music by Schoenberg and Webern, insofar as it expressly grapples with the stigmatizing deformity of asymmetry, becomes an artistic means for arousing and channeling anxiety about disability. The musical body, like the human body, is a fragile thing. The tonal musical body is particularly subject to puncture wounds—the diatonic container is permeable, and subject to chromatic intrusions. The atonal musical body is subject to the impairment of mobility, the imperiling of balance, and to deforming asymmetries. In this sense, disability and anxiety about disability appear to be central to musical modernism, at least in its Viennese atonal variety.

It is a historical irony that Schoenberg and Webern's atonal music was written at a time when people with actual deformities, disfigurations, and mobility

---

embraces beauty that seems by traditional standards to be broken, and yet it is not less beautiful but more so, as a result (2-3)....To what concept, other than the idea of disability, might be referred modern art's love affair with misshapen and twisted bodies, stunning variety of human forms, intense representation of traumatic injury and psychological alienation, and unyielding preoccupation with wounds and tormented flesh? (4).

See also Nochlin 1994.

impairments had been rendered largely invisible by institutions designed to serve and simultaneously sequester them (Stiker 2000). Neither composer had any direct experience with physical disability, nor was it a prominent part of their world, apart from aestheticized representations of the grotesque in the arts. Their music encodes and responds to an anxiety about disability, but does so largely in the abstract.

Amid the Great War and its immediate aftermath, however, Schoenberg and Webern, like all citizens of Europe, found that disability had become a pervasive part of their daily lives. Suddenly, the streets of Vienna (like those of other European capitals) were full of wounded war veterans with physical impairments and deformities of all kinds. And, amid the economic chaos that attended the end of the war, the effects of poverty and starvation on the bodies of their fellow citizens, particularly children, would have been unavoidable as well.[9]

In the same period, during and immediately after the war, both Schoenberg and Webern fell silent as composers. Their prewar music had been concerned to some degree with representations of the human body, and with narratives of bodily disability. Perhaps their silence was due, in part, to their search for an appropriate artistic response to a new sense of the human body, one sharply influenced by direct experience of disability on a large scale. Some contemporary visual artists, such as George Grosz and Otto Dix, responded with direct representations of those wounded in the war. Schoenberg and Webern appear to have responded in precisely the opposite way. In their prewar music, disability had entered the musical body in the form of asymmetry, posing a challenge to a normative symmetry. Within these atonal works, normative symmetry once unsettled is not usually reestablished in any definitive way, and to that extent these works may be understood as accommodating bodily difference. When they resumed composing after the war, however, both composers adopted twelve-tone, serial styles that remained fundamentally concerned with inversional balance and symmetry, but approached them in a quite different way. Although the prewar music accommodated asymmetry, the postwar, twelve-tone music banished it, at least from the deeper levels of structure.

In Webern's twelve-tone music, the normative polyphonic combination involves series-forms related by inversion. Literal symmetries in register typically reinforce the underlying structural symmetry. Instead of the flexible interaction of symmetry and asymmetry typical of his free, atonal music, we find that inversional symmetry and balance permeate the entire musical fabric, from top to bottom and from beginning to end, without any serious challenge.[10] The hallmark of Schoenberg's mature twelve-tone music likewise involves combinations of series related to each

9. The extensive disability, deformity, and disfigurement brought about by the Great War and its immediate aftermath have been thoroughly documented. See Whalen (1984), Boyer (1995), Gerber (2000), Cohen (2001), and Healy (2004).

10. For one among many published descriptions of the role of inversional symmetry in Webern's twelve-tone music, see Bailey (1991).

other by inversion.[11] In Schoenberg's twelve-tone music, the surface is often asymmetrical in striking ways, but the inversional symmetry of the underlying twelve-tone structure is guaranteed in advance.[12]

The dramatic shift in the social and visual landscape of wartime and postwar Vienna may have been among the factors that gave rise to the twelve-tone idea, which, for Schoenberg and Webern, is fundamentally concerned with inversional balance and symmetry. As one of its central achievements, the "method of composing with twelve tones" establishes a secure harmonic framework grounded in inversional symmetry and balance. Typically in a twelve-tone piece by Schoenberg or Webern, the sense of inversional balance is far more pervasive and far more stable than in their atonal music. The sense of balance in their twelve-tone music is explicit, fundamental, and unimpaired.

When people with physical disabilities were largely invisible to them, Schoenberg and Webern wrote music that explored extremes of asymmetry and imbalance, and generally refused explicit solutions to the problems they posed. When people with physical disabilities become an everyday part of the visual landscape, with an attendant rise in social and cultural anxiety about disability, Schoenberg and Webern responded with a musical language that guaranteed stable balance and virtually banished the possibility of lingering asymmetry. In this sense, we can see in the twelve-tone idea an extreme avoidance reaction to the threat of deforming asymmetry and imbalance, now made shockingly real in everyday life.

11. The technical term for the procedure is *hexachordal inversional combinatoriality*, in which a series form is combined with its inversion such that "the inversion of the first six tones, the antecedent, should not produce a repetition of one of these six tones, but should bring forth the hitherto unused six tones of the chromatic scale. Thus, the consequent of the basic set, the tones 7 to 12, comprises the tones of this inversion, but, of course, in a different order" (Schoenberg 1941/1984, 225).

12. On the relationship in Schoenberg's twelve-tone music between underlying pitch-class symmetrical twelve-tone structures and their often asymmetrical realization in pitch space, see Cherlin (1991, 2007) and Peles (2004). As Peles observes,

> The system itself is also defined at so abstract a level that it need not be—and in Schoenberg's music usually is not—associated with explicit foreground symmetry, or repetition of other obvious sorts. Instead, a maximumly asymmetrical and non-repetitive surface will typically play itself out against the backdrop of a maximumly symmetrical abstract succession (61).

CHAPTER 5

Musical Narratives of the Fractured Body: Schoenberg, Stravinsky, Bartók, and Copland

LATE STYLE AND DISABILITY STYLE

If we live long enough, all of us will become disabled. The longer we live, the more we are exposed to the vicissitudes of life and, as we age, the more certain it becomes that our bodies and minds will become impaired in some degree. For many of the composers discussed in this book, their experience of disability is associated with their advancing age. For the most part, discussions of music by older composers have fallen under the rubric of what is known as "late style."[1] Music in a "late style" is presumed to have certain internal qualities (e.g., fragmentation, intimacy, nostalgia, or concision) and to be associated with certain external factors (e.g., the age of the composer, his or her proximity to and foreknowledge of death, or a sense of authorial belatedness with respect to significant predecessors). In what follows, I will argue that "late style" is usually better understood as "disability style": older composers write the way they do because they are narrating their fractured minds and bodies. The musical stories they tell are stories of disability.

The generally accepted biographical markers of the late style turn out, on close inspection, to have less impact than disability. The age at which a composer may write "late" works varies considerably. Mozart began composing his late works (beginning with the last three symphonies in 1788) when he was thirty-three years old, whereas Schubert was only twenty-nine when he wrote the two piano trios, the final piano sonatas, and the string quintet. Even composers who are thought of as

---

1. The "late style" is a longstanding aesthetic category in all of the arts. In music, Said (2006), who draws extensively on Adorno (2002), has been the catalyst for recent discussions of the late style.

having lived into old age often initiated their distinctive late style when relatively young, at least by modern standards. Bach was only forty-five when a creative lull in 1730 led to his adoption of then-current Italian operatic and *galant* styles and still in his early sixties when he wrote the canonic masterpieces of his final years; Beethoven was only forty-eight when he wrote the "Hammerklavier" Sonata, Op. 106; and Brahms was only fifty when he wrote his Third Symphony, often described as the gateway to his late style.[2]

Superficially, it might seem that "late style" would be more reliably, even tautologically, correlated with proximity to a composer's death: late works are simply those written late in the composer's life, however long that life is. The idea appears to be that proximity to death brings special knowledge that informs the music and leads to a distinctive late style.[3] But this is problematic too. People at any age are generally unaware in advance that they are going to die; the closeness of death is known only retrospectively and only to others. Some composers certainly had vivid foreknowledge of their imminent mortality as they were writing their last works (Schubert and Bartók come immediately to mind), but that is not generally the case. Composers may have intimations of mortality at various times in their lives, perhaps more often as they age, but there is little reason to imagine that most works generally understood as being in a late style are informed in any particular way by an awareness of approaching death.[4]

For some composers, late style is associated with a sense of authorial belatedness, a feeling of having been born too late, when everything worth saying has already been said.[5] But although anxiety with respect to the towering achievements of one's predecessors seems to affect writers back almost to the invention of the written word, it comes much later to composers. In music at least, authorial belatedness and late style seem to have only a tenuous relationship.

Music written in an apparently "late style" usually has more to do with the physical and mental condition of the composer than with chronological age, proximity to death, or authorial belatedness. Most composers who write in what is recognized as a late style have shared experiences of nonnormative bodily or mental function, impairment, or disability. A list of composers whose distinctive late styles

2. On Bach, see Marshall (1976). On Brahms, see Notley (2007). The literature on Beethoven was surveyed in chapters 1 and 2.

3. See, for example, Burnham (2006): "The word 'late' names various relations to time and commands a range of connotations that begin and end in an awareness of death. This awareness figures heavily into how we construe lateness and late works." Likewise, see Updike (2006): "Yet, at least for this aging reader, works written late in a writer's life retain a fascination. They exist, as do last words, where life edges into death, and perhaps have something uncanny to tell us."

4. As Micznik (1996, 163) observes, "The equation between late style and death depends on mythologizing techniques rather than stylistic arguments."

5. The work of Harold Bloom is the principal source for discussions of authorial belatedness (Bloom 1973, 1975, 1976, 1983). For Bloom-inspired discussions of music, see Straus (1990) and Korsyn (1991).

were coincident with disability (including physical and mental impairments resulting from disease or other causes) would include many discussed already in this book—Delius (blindness), Beethoven and Smetana (deafness), Schumann and possibly Ravel (madness)—as well as many others, including Bach (blindness), Tchaikovsky (various health problems), Mahler (heart condition), Debussy (rectal cancer), Bartók (leukemia), Schoenberg (heart condition and other health problems), Stravinsky (stroke), and Copland (Alzheimer's disease). In such cases, the experience of living with a disability is a more potent impetus for late-style composition than age, foreknowledge of death, or authorial belatedness. In this reading, late style may be less about anticipating death than living with a disability, less about a hypothetical future than the present reality.

Just as composers may have different experiences of disability and may respond to that experience in different ways, critics have identified a variety of characteristics of what they call the late style. Nonetheless, a survey of the vast literature on the late works of major composers will find a surprising degree of unanimity about the qualities of the musical style.[6] These qualities can be distilled into six reasonably distinct categories or clusters of adjectives, all drawn from the published literature on a large group of canonical composers (for each cluster I have selected one adjective to name the category and stand for the rest).

- *Introspective.* Alienated, apart, detached, estranged, exiled, intimate, introverted, isolated, personal, private, refined, reflective, uncommunicative, withdrawn.
- *Austere.* Anonymous, bare, elemental, expressionless, immobilized, impersonal, laconic, objective, pared down, rarefied, restrained, simple, spare, stripped down.
- *Difficult.* Abstract, bitter, catastrophic, complex, contradictory, contrapuntal (canonic), enigmatic, experimental, formidable, incomprehensible, intransigent, irascible, mannerist, technically advanced, tense, severe, socially resistant, spiny, unconcerned about pleasing.
- *Compressed.* Compact, concentrated, concise, condensed, dense, distilled, economical, miniaturized, pithy, unadorned, undecorated, unencumbered, unornamented.
- *Fragmentary.* Attenuated, discontinuous, episodic, fissured, furrowed, heterogeneous, interrupted, juxtaposed, loosely structured, nonharmonious, paratactic, ravaged, riven, torn, unintegrated, unreconciled.
- *Retrospective.* Anachronistic, archaic, fascinated with the past, lucid, lyrical, naïve, nostalgic, serene, simplified, spiritual, translucent.

A list of this kind is necessarily crude. On the one hand, the categories overlap to some extent; on the other, they occasionally seem to contradict each other: music written in the late style is difficult and simple, expressionless and intimately communicative, ahead of its time and retrospective in character, diffuse and compressed.

6. Straus (2008) offers such a survey.

In response, we might attempt to understand late style as descriptive of a group of works that share at least some of these characteristics, but not necessarily all of them. We might wish to speak of late styles (in the plural), with variations depending on the composer and the work and, to a significant extent, on the temperament and interests of the critic. It would be unlikely for any single work to share all of these characteristics, but a late-style work would necessarily have most of them. Or, we might imagine that works in a late style simply involve certain internal contradictions—the inherent tension among these different characteristics is itself a marker of stylistic lateness.

These metaphors of late style largely involve ascriptions to musical works of bodily or mental states. Specifically, the characteristics associated with the late style are largely evocative of disabled or impaired bodies or minds and their failure to function in a normal way. Many of the characteristics of late style suggest nonnormative physical, mental, or emotional states, and even specific "disorders" such as autism (detached, estranged from reality, isolated, socially resistant), depression (expressionless, laconic, immobilized), schizophrenia (torn, fissured, nonharmonious, fragmentary), senile dementia (backward-looking, simplified), mobility impairments (immobilized), or general physical disintegration (fractured, furrowed, fissured).

Although this kind of criticism might be dismissed as pathologizing a style, treating it as deviant and abnormal with respect to the mature style that precedes it and thus practicing criticism as a form of diagnosis, I would prefer to see a deeper truth in these metaphors: *late style works are those that represent nonnormative mental and bodily states.* The disabilities of their composers are refracted into a general sense of nonnormative bodily or mental function and inscribed in their music. That inscription then gives rise to the aesthetic category of the late style. Thus, both the music and the discourse about it position disability at the center of the late style.

To illustrate this contention, I offer disability-inflected readings of four late-style works by four twentieth-century modernist composers: Stravinsky's *Requiem Canticles;* Schoenberg's String Trio; Bartók's Third Piano Concerto; and Copland's *Night Thoughts.* Biographical information links all four works explicitly with the deteriorating bodily condition of the composer. I will argue that, at least in these works, *late style is disability style.*

STRAVINSKY, *REQUIEM CANTICLES*

Requiem Canticles (1966) is Stravinsky's last major work. Written at a time of deteriorating health, it is self-evidently a personal work, as Stravinsky's wife, Vera, has confirmed: "*He* and *we* knew he was writing it for himself" (quoted in Craft 1972/1994, 376–77). Robert Craft, Stravinsky's amanuensis during his final twenty years, has suggested that it was designed as a memorial to friends recently deceased:

The sketch book of the *Requiem Canticles* is also a necrology of friends who died during its composition. The composer once referred to these pasted-in obituaries as a "practical commentary." Each movement seems to relate to an individual death, and though Stravinsky denies that it really does, the framing of his musical thoughts by the graves of friends (that touching cross for Giacometti) exposes an almost unbearably personal glimpse of his mind (Craft 1972/1994, 309).[7]

The work is deeply engaged with all six of the metaphorical markers of the late style identified above. First, it is introspective and emotionally restrained. Its small instrumental forces, often used in chamber-music fashion, give it an intimate, private aspect, particularly in comparison with other requiem masses in the music literature. Second, it is austere—as radically stripped down and emotionally undemonstrative as anything Stravinsky ever wrote. Third, it is difficult in its highly advanced musical language, involving Stravinsky's own distinctive adaptation of the twelve-tone method of Schoenberg, Webern, and Krenek.[8] Although there are many homophonic, chorale-like passages, the music is deeply contrapuntal and canonic, down to the basic construction of the "rotational arrays" on which it is based. Fourth, it is highly compressed, concise, and economical. There is no filler, no ornamentation—every detail seems to carry structural weight. The text is stripped down and stated directly, without repetition; the whole work, made up of nine brief movements, can be performed in under fifteen minutes. Fifth, there is a strong sense of fragmentation, of a musical whole that has been blown into discrete bits that are barely held together. Stravinsky's music, both early and late, often gives the impression of an assemblage of discrete units. It sounds, in many cases, as though discrete textural blocks have been cut out and pasted together, and that is sometimes literally true.[9] But the fragmentation is particularly intense in *Requiem Canticles,* and is reinforced by two other recurring characteristics of Stravinsky's style, particularly in his late music: extended silences and musical "stuttering," that is, the oscillation between two melodic notes or two harmonies. Sixth, it has a strongly retrospective character in several respects. As Taruskin (1996, 1650) notes, in its evocation of tolling bells, religious

---

7. See also Walsh (2006, 523):

> Like the *Introitus,* but unlike his other memorial pieces, Stravinsky wrote [*Requiem Canticles*] in a specifically elegiac spirit, pasting into the sketchbook as he went along obituaries of friends who died during its composition—an extraordinary reversal of his habitual refusal to associate his work with current events or feelings.

8. For a description of the technical features of Stravinsky's late, serial music, see Straus (2001).

9. Nabokov (1951, 152) quotes Stravinsky's account of using scissors and paste in composing *Orpheus.* This feature of Stravinsky's music has been widely acknowledged. See, for example, Van den Toorn (1983, 454), where the phenomenon, termed "block juxtaposition," is identified as a "peculiarly Stravinskian conception of form." Taruskin (1996, 1677) calls this feature *Drobnost,* defined as "splinteredness; the quality of being formally disunified, a sum-of-parts," and identifies it as one of Stravinsky's most basic style characteristics.

chorales, and Russian Orthodox liturgical music, "the piece fairly reeks with nostalgia." The narrative arc of the work, and its expressive impact, depend on a basic contrast between formations with and without traditional diatonic reference. Although the work is strictly twelve-tone in conception—every note in the work, without exception, can be traced to underlying twelve-tone arrays—it nonetheless seems at times to recall a more traditionally consonant, diatonic state.

All six of these late-style characteristics may be related to the increasingly difficult physical circumstances of Stravinsky's old age.[10] The last two in particular—fragmentation and retrospection—bear a particularly important relationship to Stravinsky's bodily condition. The fragmented musical surface of *Requiem Canticles*, with its discrete, isolated textural blocks, may be heard as a metaphorical recreation of physical disintegration, of a body fracturing and losing its organic wholeness. The retrospective qualities of the music, particularly at the beginning and end of the work, give a sense of a descent into a world of struggle, of physical obstacles, impediments, and impairments, and a partial and ambiguous attempt at recuperation through a return to a prior normal state.

In the opening measures of the Prelude to *Requiem Canticles*, an accompanying chord in steady sixteenth notes is built up, one note at a time: F-C-B-A. The texture is then reduced to A alone, which moves to D at the end of the passage. These five notes are obviously diatonic in character, and one of the things that *Requiem Canticles* is about is an attempt to reattain at its end the simple, open, white-note quality of this beginning.

The melody offers significant contrast, tracing six different notes grouped in pairs: A-sharp–C, D-A, G–C-sharp. The first of those pairs involves a three-fold repetition of the kind Stravinsky refers to as a "stutter": "two reiterated notes [which] are a melodic-rhythmic stutter characteristic of my speech from *Les Noces* to the *Concerto in D*, and earlier and later as well—a lifelong affliction, in fact" (Stravinsky and Craft 1966, 58).[11] This melodic gesture is often associated with grief, or with a kind of somber muteness in the face of death.

10. As Craft and Vera Stravinsky observe,

    Like other artists in their eighties who continue to create (and not just to produce), Stravinsky's sense of isolation increased, the ferocity of his impatience grew, and his *saeva indignatio* [savage indignation] kindled more quickly. Like that of some others, too, his art of these years is marked by a greater concentration—spareness, severity—and by a tendency to sacrifice surface attractions to structural ideas (V. Stravinsky and Craft 1978, 486).

11. Stravinsky makes this observation with reference to the alternation of the notes D and E in the vocal line of *Elegy for J. F. K.* to set the words, "The Heavens are silent." Van den Toorn (1983, 440) relates the "melodic-rhythmic stutter" to Stravinsky's persistent predilection for musical oscillations of all kinds: "The 'two reiterated notes' are ultimately a form of back-and-forth oscillation; and in this respect they may indeed be found reaching into every crevice of melodic, rhythmic, formal, or pitch-relational matter." Jers (1976) contains a useful list and discussion of melodic stutters in Stravinsky's late music.

In *Requiem Canticles* the melodic stutter seems to convey a sense of self-enclosure, of inescapable circularity, and of forced acquiescence in an incomprehensible fate. The melodic stutter, with its alternation of notes a whole tone apart, is reinforced by a similar harmonic stutter: the first harmony of the passage is transposed up a whole-tone to become the last harmony of the passage. Both harmonic and melodic stutters reinforce the sense of this passage as a discrete block, a fragment separated by silence from other fragments.

In all of this, we have a sense of a physical body that is not functioning normally. The stutter in Stravinsky's music, as in real life, suggests an inability to speak fluently.[12] That apparent disfluency renders the melody static, fixed in place, and enhances the isolation of the musical fragment of which it is part. And the fragmentation of lines within the textural block—and of the textural block in relation to other blocks—also suggests a physical body that is immobilized and falling to pieces. To some extent, the rest of *Requiem Canticles* can be understood to be an effort, ultimately only partially successful at best, to return to the unimpaired diatonicism of the opening, to transcend the pervasive fragmentation, and to recuperate a sense of physical wholeness.

The Postlude from *Requiem Canticles,* the final movement of the work, consists of three distinct and separately evolving musical strands. The first involves three twelve-chord chorales, scored for *celeste, campane,* and *vibraphone.* The second involves five widely spaced chords presented before, between, and after the chorales. These chords, scored for flutes, piano, harp, and French horn, have been referred to as "Chords of Death."[13] The third consists of long sustained notes in the French Horn. The three strands are distinguished by texture and instrumentation and they are usually separated by silences, the longest and most profoundly expressive Stravinsky ever wrote. As in the Prelude, the stratification of the texture and the isolation of the textural blocks reinforced by silences create a sense of extreme fragmentation. This is music that moves fitfully, haltingly.

The fitful, halting motions can be understood as moving in a particular direction, namely toward a state of relative clarity and diatonicity. This is particularly evident in the progression of the five "Chords of Death," which move from large, complex, chromatic chords of five, six, seven, or eight different notes, to a relatively simple diatonic conclusion, a process of gradual simplification and clarification. The end of the Postlude therefore returns us to something like the beginning of the Prelude. One might imagine the narrative trajectory as descend-

---

12. For consideration of the musical implications of stuttering as a disability, see Goldmark (2006) and Oster (2006). On vocal disfluency generally, see Stras (2006).
13. The term "chord of death" comes from Craft (1972/1994) in his description of a performance of the *Requiem Canticles* at Stravinsky's own funeral. He describes the structure of the Postlude as "the chord of Death, followed by silence, the tolling of bells, and again silence, all thrice repeated, then the three final chords of Death alone" (415).

ing into and then emerging from a darkly rich chromatic night into a bright diatonic day.[14]

The final chord also represents a convergence of the three distinct textural strands with all three instrumental groups contributing to it. There is a sense here, however brief, that the extreme fragmentation has been overcome and a lost feeling of wholeness has been restored. Like the move toward the diatonic, however, this sense of wholeness restored—of wounds closed and healed—is fleeting and ambiguous. If one imagines the extreme fragmentation of this music, reinforced by stuttering and silence, as emblematic of a physical body that is no longer functioning normally, there can be little comfort in this ending. What we have here is not so much a cure narrative, so common in artistic representations of disability, but rather a narrative of ambivalent acceptance of a disabled condition. From this point of view, the features of the music that might usually be understood as markers of a late style, can be understood instead as expressions of and responses to disability, to the breakdown of a physical body, of the composer's own body.

SCHOENBERG, STRING TRIO

Schoenberg wrote his String Trio in the fall of 1946. At the time of its composition, Schoenberg was seventy-two years old, in increasingly poor health, living in somewhat straitened economic circumstances, and still an outsider in his adopted country. The String Trio is generally understood as typical of Schoenberg's late style, with characteristics that bring it into close conformity with late-style works generally.

First, the String Trio has a quality of intimacy and introspection. In part, this is due simply to the medium—chamber music almost inevitably entails a sense of private, personal utterance—but also to the vividness and directness of its rhetoric. The secondary literature on the String Trio has emphasized its private, inner-directed quality as emblematic of Schoenberg's late style.[15] The literature also points

14. This sense of an awakening into death recalls the scene from Tolstoy's *War and Peace* in which Prince Andrei is lying mortally wounded on his deathbed, and dreams of his own death:

> It comes in, and it is *death*. And Prince Andrei died. But in the same instant that he died, Prince Andrei remembered that he was asleep, and in the same instant that he died, he made an effort with himself and woke up. "Yes, that was death. I died—I woke up. Yes, death is an awakening." Clarity suddenly came to his soul, and the curtain that until then had concealed the unknown was raised before his inner gaze. He felt the release of a force that previously had been as if bound in him and that strange lightness which from then on did not leave him (Tolstoy 1869/2007, 985).

15. See, for example, Lessem (1997, 67): "In late works such as the String Trio and the Fantasy for Violin with piano accompaniment, we find a retreat from the greater classicizing ambition of the first mature twelve-tone works and a return to the pithy, aphoristic, loosely structured manner of pre–World War I expressionism." Likewise, see Rubsamen (1951, 481–82):

frequently to other familiar late-style characteristics in the String Trio, including difficulty in comprehension arising from extreme compression.[16]

Beyond its intimacy, compression, and difficulty, the String Trio has been widely noted for its retrospective character (another familiar late-style characteristic). Specifically, it overtly engages aspects of traditional tonality in ways that Schoenberg's mature style (the pre-late music) generally avoids.[17] In addition to its tonal reminiscences, the Trio is retrospective in another sense. The work is in five parts, with its three "Principal Sections" separated by two "Episodes," and the last Principal Section is a modified recapitulation of the first. Nearly literal recapitulations of this kind are virtually unknown in Schoenberg's music and, indeed, Schoenberg argued against them.[18] The programmatic justification and significance of the recapitulation

---

The String Trio marks the beginning of Schoenberg's last phase, during which he wrote more introspectively and intimately than before. Whereas the *Ode to Napoleon* and the Variations for Band seem to have been dedicated to a more general public, and have a more direct appeal, these last compositions are more abstract, compact, and difficult to comprehend. One looks in vain for the clear thematic construction of the earlier twelve-tone works—here the ideas are more fragmentary and hard to follow, owing to Schoenberg's emphasis upon brevity, requiring the condensation of ideas to the point of close juxtaposition and even simultaneity.

16. As Haimo (1998, 168–69) observes,

The Trio has long been regarded as one of the most complicated of Schoenberg's twelve-tone works. To the listener, particularly the first-time listener, the surface of the Trio presents numerous challenges to easy comprehensibility....At the same time, the Trio has challenged many theorists, who have found its twelve-tone structures difficult to follow.

17. See, again, Haimo (1998, 175):

Although its references to tonal elements are far more restrained than those of the Ode [to Napoleon], the Trio is by no means devoid of such references. And certainly by comparison with the twelve-tone works of the 1930s, where tonal references were studiously avoided, the Trio is quite obvious in its willingness to employ tonal elements....Although the Trio is unique, it shares many essential characteristics with other of Schoenberg's late twelve-tone works: the treatment of the source hexachord as the fundamental building block of musical structure, the pervasive use of symmetrical relationships, both pitch and order number, and the unabashed willingness to try to interleave elements of tonal syntax into the context of a twelve-tone serial composition.

Likewise, see Rosen (1975, 95): "Like many of his later works, [the Trio] is based on a series that permits the introduction of the perfect triads associated with tonality, although it avoids any implication of the harmonic function of tonality. Schoenberg uses these perfect triads for what might be called their latent aspects of sweetness and repose."

18. See Bailey (1984, 156), which offers a pertinent account by Leonard Stein, Schoenberg's longtime assistant:

Perhaps the most significant of Stein's reminiscences concerns the very unusual recapitulation section of the Trio. Part Three of the work is a nearly literal recapitulation of earlier portions of the composition, a procedure which Schoenberg had spoken out against in his writings and generally avoided in his own compositions. Stein recalls that Schoenberg had often pointed out the lack of an exact recapitulation in the Second Chamber Symphony to his students, citing as a reason the axiom that "once you have lived your life you need not go back and live it again."

will be discussed below. For now, it suffices to observe that it enhances the retrospective quality of the Trio, a work concerned with recalling not only older tonal prototypes, but also earlier parts of itself.

The late-style characteristic most dramatically in evidence in Schoenberg's String Trio is that of fragmentation. And, as Cherlin observes, its extreme fragmentation is bound up with its compressed and retrospective qualities:

> The Trio is extraordinary in the degree to which extreme contrasts and even apparent *non sequiturs* seem to fracture its surface. The music is full of abrupt and striking changes of texture and affect as musical ideas are broken off, interrupted by other ideas that are themselves interrupted in turn. But the discontinuities of the work's surface go beyond the juxtaposition of conflicting affects, disruptions, and *non sequiturs*. In surprising ways the Trio seems alternately to remember and then abandon the musical languages of its historical antecedents. Passages that employ harsh, strident dissonance give way to ones that evoke the sweetness of tonality, only to reemerge and begin the process again (Cherlin 1998, 559).[19]

In all of these ways, then—introspection, compression, difficulty, retrospection, and fragmentation—the String Trio exemplifies what is generally thought of as late style. One might imagine relating these characteristics to various aspects of Schoenberg's life and circumstances—his advancing age, his sense of alienation in the United States, his nostalgia for the musical past—but a readier explanation lies close at hand. The String Trio is essentially a programmatic work, and the program it embodies involves the story of what Schoenberg referred to as his *Todesfall* (decease), that is, his near-death experience on August 2, 1946, and his recovery from it. All of the late-style characteristics of the music serve to express this dramatic program.

In this sense, the music is not so much about lateness, in any sense, as it is about a profound experience of disability. Schoenberg not only represents disability programmatically in the music but also recreates musically the most common disability narrative, namely the cure narrative. As discussed in chapter 2, in Western literature since the late eighteenth century, narratives that engage disability typically move from a state of health or normality, through a state of illness or abnormality, to a final state of health or normality regained—a narrative of overcoming or cure. The narrative in Schoenberg's String Trio begins

---

19. Cherlin (1998, 581) brings Beethoven into the picture:

> Its fractured rhetoric, halting broken phrases, and seeming inability to settle into an even relatively stable musical space do have a predecessor in Beethoven.... It is in his late works that this particular aspect of Beethovenian rhetoric becomes exaggerated.... And of course the association of these works with grave illness toward the end of the composer's life is well known.

As Cherlin suggests, the late styles of Beethoven and Schoenberg are associated with each other and with their shared experience of disability.

somewhere in the middle of this larger trajectory, but strongly emphasizes the sense of restoration at its end.

The following is a chronological account of the Schoenberg's *Todesfall*.[20] On August 2, 1946, a Dr. Waitzfelder arrived at Schoenberg's house in Los Angeles late in the morning. He examined Schoenberg and prescribed a pill for Schoenberg's asthma, a new drug called Benzedrine (an amphetamine). During lunch, Schoenberg felt extremely tired and his wife, Gertrude, put him to bed and he slept until 9:30 P.M. He then awoke suddenly "with an extremely unpleasant feeling, but without definite pain" and hurried to his armchair. He started to feel worse—"A very heavy pain started at once in my whole body, especially in the chest and around the heart"—and had his wife call Leonard Stein, his assistant. Stein arrived shortly thereafter with a Dr. Lloyd Jones. Jones determined that Schoenberg was not having a heart attack, but nonetheless administered an injection of Dilaudid (a pain medication). In Schoenberg's words, "It worked very quickly. The pain went away. Then I must have lost consciousness.... After ten minutes I lost consciousness, had no heart beat or pulse and stopped breathing. In other words, I was practically dead."

Jones, Stein, and Schoenberg's wife carried him to bed where he lay unconscious for several hours. During the period of unconsciousness, Schoenberg was delirious. Schoenberg's wife reported that, "We worked with adrenalin, oxygen and hot water bottles till five in the morning. In the early morning things had gone so far that he wanted to get up. He didn't know anything about his whole collapse. The cardiogram showed an irregular rhythm but no heart attack."[21]

Schoenberg himself had no personal memory of the delirium or the efforts made on his behalf while he was unconscious. When he finally regained consciousness in the morning of the next day, he reported that "The first thing I remember was that a man with coal-black hair was bending over me and making every effort to feed me something.... It was Gene, the male nurse. An enormous person, a former boxer, who could pick me up and put me down again like a sofa cushion."

It took Schoenberg roughly three weeks to recover from this incident, during which time he stayed upstairs in his bedroom. Doctors attended him there and, among other treatments, administered numerous injections of penicillin (it is hard not to wonder about the quality of the medical care that Schoenberg received

20. Schoenberg offered several different accounts of the experience, and additional details were provided by his wife and students. Relevant documents are reprinted in Auner (2003) and Bailey (1984).

21. It should be emphasized that here and throughout his accounts of the episode, Schoenberg affirms that whatever the source of his sudden illness, it was not a heart attack. The secondary literature nonetheless virtually always assumes a heart attack. It seems more likely that Schoenberg was, in fact, experiencing a strong reaction to Dilaudid.

throughout this episode). During this period of convalescence, Schoenberg wrote the bulk of his String Trio. The final section, the modified recapitulation mentioned above, was completed when he finally felt well enough to return to his studio downstairs.

Schoenberg referred to the Trio as a "'humorous' representation of my sickness"[22] and affirmed in conversations with students and friends that it embodied his experience of illness, near death, and recovery. The best-known account of the link between the Trio and the *Todesfall* is Thomas Mann's:

> [Schoenberg] told me about the new trio he had just completed, and about the experiences he had secretly woven into the composition—experiences of which the work was a kind of fruit. He had, he said, represented his illness and medical treatment in the music, including even the male nurses and all the other oddities of American hospitals.[23]

Schoenberg's students Hanns Eisler, Leonard Stein, and Adolf Weiss all reported that Schoenberg claimed to have represented aspects of his illness and recovery in the String Trio (Bailey 1984; Rubsamen 1951).

The precise nature of the relationship between Schoenberg's illness and the music, however, is a matter of considerable confusion and contradiction. The only programmatic elements on which there is general agreement is that certain loud chords represent injections of penicillin[24] and, much more important, that the fragmentary nature of the musical discourse reflects the agitated state of Schoenberg's mind, including his unconscious delirium:

> According to Stein, Schoenberg explained the many juxtapositions of unlike material within the Trio as reflections of the delirium which the composer suffered during parts of his illness. Thus, the seemingly fragmentary nature of the Trio's material represents the experience of time and events as perceived from a semiconscious or highly sedated state. These unusual juxtapositions also represent, as reported by Rubsamen, the alternate phases of "pain and suffering" and "peace and repose" that Schoenberg experienced (Bailey 1984, 156–57).

The opening music of the Trio is highly agitated and fragmented. I imagine that this music represents the onset of Schoenberg's illness, the moment when he awakens suddenly after a long rest, realizes he is unwell, and staggers to his armchair in growing confusion and alarm. Toward the end of part 1, the anguish seems to subside—the music becomes quieter and more continuous and the twelve-tone

---

22. Schoenberg, "My Fatality," quoted in Bailey (1984, 152).
23. Mann's account is cited in Bailey (1984, 155).
24. According to Bailey (1984, 156–57), "Another subjective feature that Stein remembers is the presence of the penicillin injections, which are represented in the score by loud and striking passages which tend to interrupt calmer sections...."

structures are expressed with relative clarity. I imagine that this change of mood reflects the confidence and relative calm inspired by the arrival of Dr. Jones, who assures Schoenberg that he has not had a heart attack. At some point, possibly represented by a *pizzicato* chord right at the end of part 1, Dr. Jones administers the injection of Dilaudid, and Schoenberg falls unconscious. The moment when Schoenberg loses consciousness is one of unusual tranquility and sweetness, with an explicit reference to an A-major triad, and possibly to the key of A major.[25] The sudden simplification of the musical texture and the tonal reminiscence reflect Schoenberg's mental state, which has moved from agitation and anguish to profound peace.

The narrative journey culminates in the modified recapitulation with which the work ends. Stein relates the recapitulation explicitly to the restoration of Schoenberg's health:

> Part three of the work is a nearly literal recapitulation of earlier portions of the composition, a procedure which Schoenberg had spoken out against in his writings and generally avoided in his own compositions.... In the case of the Trio, after the tormented and confused depiction of the portion of this life found in the first section of the work, Schoenberg felt justified in going back and "reliving" that portion with the calmness and perspective of good health. Significantly enough, Schoenberg composed the bulk of the work while he was still too ill to leave his bedroom. It was not until he reached part three of the Trio, the recapitulation, that he was able to "come downstairs" to his regular workroom (Quoted in Bailey 1984, 156–57).[26]

The Trio ends gently, with a final reminiscence of the tranquil, A-centered idea from the beginning of the first Episode. In its sense of intimacy, heightened by the singing, cantabile style, its clarity and simplicity, its recall of traditional tonal materials, this concluding music is a paradigm of the late style generally and of Schoenberg's late style more specifically. In the context of the programmatic allusions to Schoenberg's illness and the narrative trajectory of health lost and then restored—a familiar cure narrative—the concluding music speaks more of Schoenberg's bodily condition than of lateness in any sense.

25. Keller (1994, 216–17) refers to this moment as "an outbreak of tonality," describing the passage in A major, and referring to the D-sharp as "a leading-note to the dominant." Cherlin (1998) also talks about the yearning quality of D-sharp in this context.
26. Likewise, see Whittall (2001, 16):

> To constrain Part 3's progression to a "death-rebirth" scenario would be crude in the extreme, yet the fact that the music stems from, and also represents, Schoenberg's being brought back to life after a heart attack, gives particularly intensity to the point at which the two types of material [turbulent vs. tranquil] are first "confused."

As with Schoenberg, Bartók's late-period music was composed in exile in the United States amid financial insecurity and increasingly poor health.[27] Bartók settled in New York in October 1940, near the tail end of the influx of increasingly desperate émigrés and refugees from war-torn Europe. During his American years, cut short by his death in 1945 at the age of sixty-four, he supported himself primarily through ethnographical work at Columbia University and concert tours as a pianist or duo-pianist (with his wife). His financial situation was precarious and a source of constant anxiety.[28] More serious, Bartók's health began to deteriorate not long after his arrival. He was diagnosed with leukemia in April 1942 and the disease reached a critical stage in February 1943, when Bartók was hospitalized for a time.[29]

During his difficult American years, Bartók composed only four works: the Concerto for Orchestra (1943), the Sonata for Solo Violin (1944), Piano Concerto No. 3 (1945), and Viola Concerto (1945). The Concerto for Orchestra was written in the summer of 1943 in a sanatorium at Saranac Lake, New York, where Bartók was attempting to recuperate, and was experiencing somewhat improved health. The Sonata for Solo Violin was written in another sanatorium, this one in Asheville, North Carolina, again during a period of relatively good health. The Piano Concerto No. 3 and Viola Concerto were written simultaneously during a final period of declining health, and the Viola Concerto was left unfinished at his death.

27. The following biographical sketch is based on Stevens (1993), Tallián (1995), and Gillies (2001).

28. There is debate in the literature about the extent of Bartók's financial need. Tallián (1995, 102) argues that,

> Bartók was traumatized by his new environment, so different from the one he had been accustomed to for sixty years. His position in relation to his environment was also different from what it had been, beyond comparison.... In America he had neither a job with retirement benefits nor a central place in cultural life as its greatest hero. As a result, he was forced literally to struggle for his existence. He found himself, at sixty, in a state of insecurity equal to or even greater than that during his greatest previous crisis, endured between 1904 and 1906, before his appointment to the Conservatory.

> Gillies (2001, 200) counters that, "With hindsight it is possible to say that the claims of poverty were exaggerated. Yet as life is lived forwards, rather than backwards, Bartók's anxieties—and with them, a widespread impression of destitution—are easily understandable."

29. As Gillies (2001, 198) recounts,

> By April 1942 his leukemia had been tentatively diagnosed, although the exact nature of the disease appears to have been held back from Bartók. His health only became critical in late February 1943, shortly after he had started presenting lectures at Harvard University. He was hospitalized—his weight had dropped to an alarming 40 kilograms [88 pounds]—and intensive investigations of his condition were undertaken. Hence, through the mediation of Hungarian friends, ASCAP took over management of his case, and in the following two-and-a-half years reportedly spent about $16,000 on his medical care and several periods of recuperation at Saranac Lake, New York, and Asheville, North Carolina.... What is now clear is that Bartók was ill during the entirety of his American years with progressive stages of blood disorders.

All four works are described in the critical literature as sharing certain familiar late-style characteristics, including especially those clustering in my sixth category: retrospection, anachronism, archaism, nostalgia, and simplification. These characteristics are particularly pronounced in the Third Piano Concerto, according to Stevens (1993):

> The serenity of the Third Piano Concerto is remarkable among Bartók's larger works.... His progressive trend toward both structural and tonal lucidity is exemplified through the Third Piano Concerto. In both texture and orchestration there is extreme clarity, sometimes to the point of tenuousness (250)....If the Third Piano Concerto is to be considered weaker than the first two, it must be because of the extreme refinement of its idiom (252)....Both the harmonic and the melodic elements of the Concerto represent a distillation of Bartók's maturest style: the tendency toward a more strongly affirmed tonality, lucid textures, plastic rhythms, is here intensified (280).

The opening of the second movement of the Third Piano Concerto would seem to exemplify Bartók's late-style interest in simplicity and lucidity, not to mention another familiar late-style interest: imitative counterpoint.

As the movement begins, the strings present a series of imitative entries, and the music confines itself to the diatonic white notes. In measure 15, the first section of the movement concludes with a strange, distant, menacing intrusion of E-flat–D-flat, the two lowest and softest notes heard thus far. These notes are shockingly distant from the prevailing white-note collection, and suggest a basic dichotomy in the music, between white-note music (especially oriented toward the white-note pentatonic collections, [C, D, E, G, A] and [F, G, A, C, D]) and black-note music (especially oriented toward the black-note pentatonic collection, [G-flat, A-flat, B-flat, D-flat, E-flat]). The strangely intrusive E-flat and D-flat of measure 15 prefigure this essential black-white dichotomy and set in motion a musical narrative in which the controlling white-note pentatonic is increasingly under challenge, and almost overthrown. This musical narrative gives expression to a version of the disability-related cure narrative, one in which the final-stage restoration of health and bodily normality is ambiguous at best.

As part of its disability-related program, the music makes obvious reference to the slow movement of Beethoven's String Quartet Op. 132, a resemblance that has been noted many times (Bónis 1963; Straus 1990). Beethoven entitled that movement "a hymn of Thanksgiving to God from a convalescent, in the Lydian mode." The religious aura of Beethoven's "hymn" is enhanced by the deliberate archaism (Lydian mode) of its setting, and this is a distinctive aspect of his late style (Brandenburg 1982). Bartók's music involves an intensification of this late-style archaism, alluding both to Beethoven and, through him, to the much older precedents on which Beethoven draws. In Beethoven's quartet, the phrases of a homophonic chorale are interspersed with imitative interludes; Bartók's concerto unfolds the same way, with imitative passages in the strings interspersed with a homophonic chorale in the solo piano. The resemblance between the passages extends to their motives, rhythm, tempo, and general character.

There is also an important programmatic link between the works. Bartók's has no title, but in adopting Beethoven's manner, he simultaneously adopts Beethoven's matter, and this movement of his Third Piano Concerto is also best understood as a hymn of thanksgiving from a convalescent. The musical narrative unfolds somewhat differently in the two works, however. Beethoven's hymn alternates with a more vigorous contrasting section that Beethoven titles "Feeling new strength," and the hymn itself intensifies and deepens emotionally in each of its appearances. In the Bartók, the contrasting music gives little sense of new strength, and the final return of the opening hymn is ambiguous in its impact. If Beethoven's string quartet is a profoundly sincere offering of thanks from a convalescent who has fully recovered from an illness, Bartók's piano concerto is much more equivocal—the thanks are qualified and the recovery incomplete.

This programmatic ambiguity is felt most in the contrast between white-note and black-note diatonicism, referred to above. In the first section, with its alternation of homophonic hymn in the piano and imitative interludes in the strings, the intrusive E-flat–D-flat of measure 15 signals a gradual move toward the flat side, and the music becomes increasingly clotted with chromaticism. After a contrasting middle section that features explicit contrast and juxtaposition of white-note and black-note pentatonic formations, the opening hymn returns and reenacts the move toward the flat side. This time, however, the move to the flat side seems definitive, and the music seems to be ending on an E-flat minor triad within a black-note pentatonic environment, one that conspicuously features the problematic E-flat and D-flat from measure 15. Only a last minute diversion at the very end prevents this apparent musical disaster from taking place. But far from a definitive return to the white-note opening, the ending sounds inconclusive and equivocal at best.

Bartók's personal, physical circumstances are mirrored in this movement and in this ending. The Third Piano Concerto was written at a time when Bartók felt well enough to compose—an improvement over a slightly earlier period—but he still knew himself to be desperately ill. Beethoven's heartfelt hymn of thanksgiving is transmuted in the Bartók into something more like relief at the temporary cessation of pain, but with the relief only partial and with no expectation that it will be more than short lived. This music may be taken as typical of Bartók's late style and of late style generally in its radical simplicity and deliberate archaism. But those same characteristics may also be understood as Bartók's musical embodiment of his own physical circumstances: he is telling a story of life with a disability.

COPLAND, *NIGHT THOUGHTS*

Aaron Copland's *Night Thoughts* (1972) begins in a state of utter simplicity, with the most basic rhythms and the clearest possible diatonic harmony (pentatonic white notes focused on a G major triad). Beginning in measure 4, however, this absolutely spare, balanced opening is occluded and overwhelmed by chromaticism. By measure 10, the chromatic aggregate of all twelve tones has been completed and the simple, almost naïve, tonal-sounding opening has been obliterated. The rest of the piece can be understood as an effort to recall this opening state, to remember it musically. A succession of musical gestures lead back toward it—we glimpse fragments of it, but it remains just out of reach. Finally, at the end of the work, the musical memory of the opening is restored, but only partially, and the piece is ultimately incapable of fully remembering its opening.

Night Thoughts is highly fragmentary in its formal organization. It consists of a series of brief musical moments, none longer than eight measures in length, which are internally coherent but strangely cut off from what comes before and after them. These brief moments generally involve a high degree of internal repetition, either direct or sequential. Many of these brief musical moments seem to strive back toward the G of the opening. It is as though the music is trying to recall something deeply familiar, but can't quite get it right. The opening G and its harmonic environment remain just out of reach, glimpsed in part but inaccessible. Each of the short episodes that comprise the work embodies a new effort to reach back toward the G, and each breaks off in disappointment and frustration.

As the end of the work approaches, the opening music is repeated, and Copland's indications in the score are "as at first" and "as before." But the process of clouding over with chromaticism begins almost immediately and never lets up. The final chords all contain G, and present a direct bass motion toward G, but nonetheless persistently obscure the G with notes foreign to the opening pentatonic collection. The final two measures of the work are extraordinarily beautiful and evocative. The opening music is heard one last time—"very distant, but clear." The memory of the opening is present, but at a distance, unattainable, almost concealed by the foreground chromaticism.

Like the other works discussed in this chapter, *Night Thoughts* can be understood in terms of a disability-related cure narrative, but handled in a particular way. In Stravinsky's *Requiem Canticles*, the final phase of the narrative—the regaining of an initial state of health and normative bodily function—is associated with a sense of transcendence and spiritual awakening. In Schoenberg's String Trio, the final phase is expressive of the gratitude of a recovering convalescent. In Bartók's Third Piano Concerto, we hear again the voice of a convalescent, but in this case the recovery appears ambiguous, unsatisfactory, incomplete. In Copland's *Night Thoughts*, one experiences only the distant, unrealized hope of recovery. In contrast to Stravinsky's sense of awakening into brightness, Copland expresses a painful experience of dissolution into darkness. All four works thus engage the same disability narrative, but inflected in individual ways.

Night Thoughts was virtually Copland's final original composition (only *Proclamation*, another short piano piece, came later).[30] The work is so strange—repetitive to the point of obsession, fragmented in its form, lacking in any of the familiar Copland stylistic markers—that it has been largely overlooked in the Copland literature. Critics who have discussed it have tended to emphasize its characteristically late-style qualities—its private, intimate tone, its fragmentation, its obsessive repetitions, the willed simplicity of its opening, and the abrasive dissonance of much of the rest of it:

> With its forlorn melodies set against the funereal sonorities, the piece creates a mood of deep melancholy. After John Kozar gave the work's European premiere in 1974, one review spoke of its "highly disturbing atmosphere." At the same time, at the very end, a lingering major triad, heard "very distant, but clear," suggests some repose (Pollack 1999, 514).

> Most critics of Copland's *oeuvre* do not believe his late work sustains the level of achievement of his middle-period music, particularly that of his ballets. Yet for many, the compositions Copland wrote after 1950, in spite of their flaws, confirm his vital musical imagination still at work. In *Night Thoughts*, for example, while a three-note motive does unify the work as a whole, the material does not support the kind of emotional energy Copland evidently believed the piece contained. Not much lyricism envelops the bare linear passage marked "simply singing"; nor does the passage marked "eloquently" support that wish either. Instead, obsessive reiterations of chords and piano figurations, ranging over the extremes of the piano, are repeated over and over again. This suggests Copland's own inner preoccupations, perhaps with decline and death. Thus the piece projects a haunting atmosphere of private contemplative candor, as if clues to the beyond could be found in overtones; it is an old man's work.... These late works [*Night Thoughts, Connotations, Inscape*] contain some of the most dissonant, abrasive chords he ever wrote. How often his ear gives us harmonies that speak John Donne's words: "Never send to know for whom the bell tolls; it tolls for thee" (Tick 2000, 162–63).

For Pollack and for Tick, *Night Thoughts* is about mortality and death, "an old man's work" in contemplation of his own looming demise.

30. According to Copland and Perlis (1989, 259–60),

> *Night Thoughts* was composed for the Van Cliburn Competition (1972). It was to be played by each contestant in the 1973 Quadrenniel Competition of Fort Worth, Texas. While not a virtuosic work, *Night Thoughts* presented certain difficulties for the three hundred entrants in the composition who were required to sight-read it: unusual chords, wide spacings, and some complicated pedaling. Copland said, "My intention was to test the musicality and the ability of a performer to give coherence to a free musical form." The subtitle, *Homage to Ives*, was added after the music was composed. According to Copland, "This has not prevented performers and critics from finding Ivesian allusions in the music." (A horncall question at the beginning of the piece has been pointed to as reminiscent of *The Unanswered Question*.)

But in fact Copland was not particularly old when he wrote *Night Thoughts* and was physically in good health.[31] In 1972, Copland had a more pressing concern than his hypothetical and remote mortality: he was experiencing the memory loss associated with the early stages of dementia, presumably Alzheimer's disease.[32] Copland stopped composing around this time, most likely because his mental condition made it difficult for him to continue. Noting that "aside from these few late piano pieces and some arrangements, Copland produced no new score in the last seventeen years of his life," Pollack asserts, "That the creative output of an elderly person—especially someone on the brink of senile dementia—should taper off hardly seems cause for surprise" (Pollack 1999, 516).[33]

Although Pollack dates Copland's memory loss to the mid- or late-1970s, there is evidence that it may have begun earlier—see, for example, a letter from Copland to Nadia Boulanger in November 26, 1972, right around the time he was completing *Night Thoughts:* "I hope soon to get started on an autobiography, mostly in order to tell the story of the development of American music as I saw it in the years '20 to '50. How I wish my memory were better than it is! But I hope to write it for better or worse" (reprinted in Crist and Shirley [2006, 246]). Furthermore, Copland had reason to see memory loss as signaling a potentially serious disability. As Pollack points out, "His loss of memory scared him, because his father and his sister Laurine had both succumbed to dementia in their later years, a fate he hoped he would be spared. He consulted specialists—one doctor prescribed vitamins—but nothing really could be done" (Pollack 1999, 543).

Copland scholarship has generally shied away from discussions of his late-life dementia and has ignored the possibility that it may have played a role in the composition of his final works.[34] But the internal evidence of *Night Thoughts* suggests

31. According to actuarial tables, a 72-year old white man in the United States in 1972 could expect to live another decade, and Copland actually lived another eighteen years.

32. According to Pollack (1999, 543), "Although the symptoms resembled those of Alzheimer's, his primary physician at the time, Arnold Salop, could not a make a definitive diagnosis as to the kind of dementia he suffered from."

33. Likewise, Pollack (1999, 553) writes:

Even before Copland completed his last compositions in the early 1970s, the press reported that he had stopped composing because of some supposed antipathy toward the times. It would seem, however, that such assertions had little foundation. Copland always balanced a sharply critical view of the world with a determination to go on and do one's best. Although some clearly presumed that Copland shared their bitterness and despair, he did not. He only admitted that he had difficulty, as he entered his seventies, getting new ideas and that he would rather not compose at all than merely repeat himself. Moreover, by the mid-1970s he was experiencing memory loss. So in fact, not much time transpired between his final compositions and the onset of the dementia that afflicted his final years.

34. Lerner (2004, 335) speaks of "the still somewhat taboo topic of Copland's tragic later struggles with (presumably) Alzheimer's disease.... Perhaps just as it took time for Copland's sexual identity to be more honestly considered by the scholarly community, it will also take time for the topic of his physical and mental disabilities to be discussed openly."

that Copland was, already in 1972, thinking deeply and creatively about the loss of memory, and exploring the emotional world associated with it. *Night Thoughts* has been described as a late-style work, with its characteristic fragmentation, resistance, willed simplicity together with abrasive dissonance, and its private, introspective aura, presumably related to his contemplation of his own mortality. I suggest, on the contrary, that this work is not so much about the relatively remote prospect of death as it is about the lived reality of the earliest stage of Alzheimer's disease. Copland's experience of memory loss and the emotions associated with it are thematized and embodied in the musical work. The work's apparently late-style characteristics, including its introspection, austerity, difficulty, fragmentation, and, above all, its retrospective character, all result from Copland's creative attempt to express his mental condition musically.

WRITING THE DISABLED BODY MUSICALLY

In recent years, a considerable body of literature has emerged devoted to theorizing literary embodiment and to the possibility of "writing the body." But for the most part, the bodies in question have been somewhat idealized, and the disabled body has been virtually ignored. As Lennard Davis (1995, 158) observes:

> In recent years, hundreds of texts have claimed to be rethinking the body; but the body they have been rethinking—female, black, queer—has rarely been rethought as disabled. Normalcy continues its hegemony even in progressive areas such as cultural studies—perhaps even more so in cultural studies since there the power and ability of "transgressive" bodies tend to be romanticized for complex reasons. Disabled bodies are not permitted to participate in the erotics of power, in the power of the erotic, in economies of transgression. There has been virtually no liberatory rhetoric—outside of the disability rights movement—tied to prostheses, wheelchairs, colostomy bags, canes, or leg braces.[35]

The composers discussed in this chapter are engaged in *writing the disabled body*, inscribing in their music aspects of their experience of living with a disability. The manner in which they do so has generally been understood in light of the aesthetic category of the late style, and many of the stylistic elements of their work—its introspective, austere, difficult, compressed, and fragmentary qualities—have been interpreted as markers of lateness.

35. Likewise, see Mitchell and Snyder (1997, 5):
> The current popularity of the body in critical discourse seeks to incorporate issues of race, gender, sexuality, and class while simultaneously neglecting disability. These studies share a penchant for detecting social differences as they are emblematized in corporeal aberrancies. Within this common critical methodology physical difference exemplifies the evidence of social deviance even as the constructed nature of *physicality itself* fades from view.

I have argued, however, that these works are not about age or proximity to death, but rather about the vicissitudes of the human mind and body, that is, disability. Disability has been so thoroughly stigmatized in our culture as to render it largely invisible in critical accounts. But it has been hiding in plain sight. We know that most major composers, like most human beings, have had profound experiences of disability. It should not surprise us, then, that like nationality, race, gender, and sexuality, disability may have a significant role in shaping art, including music.

What we find when we sweep away some of the romantic fantasy that has accreted around the concept of late style is that works we have become accustomed to thinking of as late are better understood in relation to their composer's experience of disability. Indeed, "lateness" is a critical fiction we have too long imposed on a particular group of musical works. It turns out that upon close inspection, these works are not late in any meaningful sense—not written when the composer was old, or near death, or in anticipation of death. To a large extent, what we have been calling late style may be better understood as disability style.

CHAPTER 6

Disability within Music-Theoretical Traditions

MUSIC THEORY AND THE NORMAL MUSICAL BODY

Previous chapters have focused on composers and their works, teasing out narratives of disability in works by composers with disabilities. In this chapter, we turn our attention to some of the ways that musical works have been studied, analyzed, and made sense of within music-theoretical traditions. To a surprising degree, these theoretical traditions are shaped by disability, both its lived reality and its associated metaphors.

The central metaphor of the music theories surveyed here is that a work of music is a human body, a living creature with form and motion, and often with blood, organs, limbs, and skin as well. This metaphor has its roots in the organicist tradition of the late eighteenth and early nineteenth centuries, but still pervades conceptualizations of music from casual listening to formal music theory. The idea that a work of music is a body gives rise to two related ideas that implicate disability. First, if a work is a body, then it might become disabled or deformed or its function might be impaired in some way. Second, if a work is a body, it might be either normal or abnormal. One of the central tasks that traditional music theory has set for itself is to distinguish between well-formed, properly functioning, normal musical bodies, and ill-formed, poorly functioning, abnormal musical bodies.

The concept of the organic is in obvious and explicit contrast to the inorganic, that is, the mechanical. To say something is organic is to say that its parts are not mechanically assembled but grow together from a shared seed or root. But there is another contrast that is inexplicit and rarely acknowledged, but nonetheless crucial, and that is to organisms that are deficient, defective, and/or disabled. Just as the concept of the normal depends on an often-unarticulated concept of the abnormal, the concept of the praiseworthy organic (i.e., the harmonious, symmetrical body) depends on the concept of the disabled organic (i.e., the deformed, disabled body). Disability is the dark and largely unexplored underside of organicism.

For Schoenberg, a principal exponent of organicism in the twentieth century, a musical work is a living organism, with blood running through it and limbs to enable its gestures and motions:

> The term *form* is used in several different senses. In an aesthetic sense, form means that a piece is *organized*: i.e., that it consists of elements functioning like those of a living *organism* (Schoenberg 1967, 1).
>
> Therefore music does not depend upon the theme. For the work of art, like every living thing, is conceived as a whole—just like a child, whose arm or leg is not conceived separately. The inspiration is not the theme, but the whole work (Schoenberg 1948/1984, 458).
>
> Thence it became clear to me that the work of art is like every other complete organism. It is so homogeneous that in every little detail it reveals its truest, inmost essence. When one cuts into any part of the human body, the same thing always comes out—blood (Schoenberg 1912, 144).

Schoenberg's explicit point in the final quotation is that a work's inmost essence, its lifeblood, is the same throughout all parts of the body. But in making that point, Schoenberg imagined that, like human bodies, musical works may be ruptured or punctured, and the body may bleed. In that sense, disfigurement and the possibility of disability are built into Schoenberg's organicist conception.[1]

When he talks about a musical work as an organism, Schoenberg seems sometimes to be thinking mainly about its form: "Because a piece of music is like an organism, its formal members, like the limbs of an organism, are differentiated and characterized by their function—such as, for example, statement and establishing, transition and bridging, contrast, elaboration, or closing" (quoted in Carpenter 1988, 39). At other times, Schoenberg seems to be thinking about the tonality of a work:

> If one presumes ... that one such body could be the tonality in a piece of music, then ... the fundamental tone would be relatively lifeless if it did not itself contain those centrifugal and centripetal forces in its overtones that make up its life and assign its organs their

---

1. Schoenberg expresses this possibility even more emphatically in his response to a request from Zemlinsky for permission to make a cut in *Pelleas und Melisande*, which Zemlinsky had conducted in Prague in February 1918:

> First and foremost: my attitude to cuts is the same as ever. I am against removing tonsils although I know one can somehow manage to go on living without arms, legs, nose, eyes, tongue, ears, etc. In my view that sort of bare survival isn't always important enough to warrant changing something in the program of the Creator who, on the great rationing day, allotted us so and so many arms, legs, ears and other organs. And so I also hold the view that a work doesn't have to live, i.e., be performed, at all costs either, not if it means losing parts of it that may even be ugly or faulty but which it was born with (Letter to Alexander von Zemlinsky, March 20, 1918 [cited in Stein 1965, 54]).

functions. It lies in its nature to allow these forces, that in it are unified and contained, to develop and strive away from each other, as it lies in their nature to do so. Thus they become limbs, thus they perform functions, thus they independently go their own ways (quoted in Carpenter 1988, 37).

In short, a musical work is metaphorically a human body, whose individual parts—its themes, harmonies, tonality, and form; its blood, skin, and limbs—are inseparable and jointly create the larger, living totality.[2]

This metaphor—that a musical work is a body, and thus susceptible to disability—undergirds much traditional music theory. Indeed, music theory has often exemplified the medical model of disability and has taken as its task the distinguishing of forms and harmonies that are normal (stable, secure, rooted in both convention and nature) from those that are abnormal. The theoretical traditions surveyed here have their roots in the mid-nineteenth century, and thus participate in two disability-related intellectual traditions. First, these traditions assume that a musical work is a human body, with life, form, and motion, and possibly with impairments as well. Second, these traditions imagine that these musical bodies are either normal or abnormal. In the embodied metaphors that have accreted around musical works, this underlying desire to sort musical bodies, to norm them statistically, is a persistent impulse.

As a result, most standard music theories are normalizing discourses: they are designed to rationalize the abnormal elements (e.g., formal anomalies or dissonant harmonies) with respect to the normal ones. One might go even farther and suggest that most standard music theories are not only normalizing discourses but also disabling discourses. Most music theories are in the business of constructing deformations and anomalies and abnormalities precisely so that they can be corrected. Music theory creates "tonal problems" in order to solve them.[3]

2. A useful summary of Schoenberg's views on this subject is provided by Neff and Carpenter in their commentary on Schoenberg (1995, 8):

> The work is an articulated whole whose parts, he says, like the organs and limbs of the living organism, exercise their specific functions in regard to both their own external effect and their mutual relationships. He distinguishes the parts of an inanimate object from limbs of a biological body: true members, that function even though they may be at rest, are found only in organisms, and unlike parts, which are actually dead, alive from event to event only through an external power, sustain their power as a result of their organic membership in a living organism. He suggests that to symbolize the construction of a musical form one might think of a living body that is whole and centrally controlled and puts forth a certain number of limbs by means of which it is capable of exercising its life-function. In music only the whole itself is that central body. The cohesive force of such a whole comes from an inner necessity. The inner force that gives the tonal body its life is the musical idea that this body presents. The central concept for Schoenberg's theory of the presentation of the musical idea is this concept of the musical organism as a tonal body, vitalized by an inner necessity, the idea it presents.

3. The notion of music theory as a disabling discourse comes from Brian Hyer (private conversation).

SOME EMBODIED METAPHORS OF MUSIC THEORY

Language about music is always and inevitably metaphorical. If metaphor is "a figure of speech in which a name or descriptive word or phrase is transferred to an object or action different from, but analogous to, that to which it is literally applicable" (*Oxford English Dictionary*), then the difference between language and music requires metaphor to bridge the divide. Even simple, everyday language about the most basic kinds of musical relationships is shot through with metaphor, although the metaphors may be so familiar as to appear natural, direct, unmediated: musical timbres are bright or dark; melodies go up and down; chords are thick or thin; rhythms are short or long—in each case, a descriptive word or phrase from the linguistic domain, usually involving physical actions or sensory experience, is transferred to the domain of musical sounds.

In the long history of writing about music, certain metaphors have come to play a central role, especially those related to the human body and to bodily experience. An important recent movement in the fields of philosophy and linguistics has focused on the concept of *embodiment*. This movement, sometimes called "experientialism," argues that we understand the world through our prior, intimate knowledge of our own bodies.[4] Music theorists have recently extended this approach to music, arguing that it creates meaning by encoding bodily experience and that listeners make sense of music in embodied terms.[5]

According to experientialism, we use our direct, concrete, physical knowledge of our own bodies as a basis for understanding the world around us; our knowledge of the world is thus embodied. As Johnson (1987, xix) argues, "Our reality is shaped by the patterns of our bodily movement, the contours of our spatial and temporal orientation, and the forms of our interaction with objects. It is never merely a matter of abstract conceptualizations and prepositional judgments." In other words, we know what we know, and derive meaning from what we experience, based on our own physicality: "Experientialism claims that conceptual structure is meaningful because it is embodied, that is, it arises from, and is tied to, our pre-conceptual bodily experiences" (Lakoff 1987, 267). Like our knowledge of the world in

4. Among the principal sources in this area are Johnson (1987), Lakoff and Johnson (1980), Lakoff (1987), and Gibbs (1994). From a radically different point of view, an important trend in postmodern theorizing of gender, race, and sexuality focuses on the body. Some representative works in this area are Wiegman (1995), Butler (1993), and Grosz (1994). Although these two approaches differ in their premises, they share a virtually complete neglect of disability as a common feature of human bodies.

5. See, for example, Brower (1997–98, 2000, 2008), Fisher and Lochhead (2002), Gur (2008), Mead (1999), Saslaw (1996, 1997–98), and Zbikowski (1997–98, 2002, 2009). In addition, a significant body of recent musicological work has approached questions of the body and embodiment from a point of view influenced by postmodern thought. See, for example, Cusick (1994) and Maus (1993), who liken works of music to fully sexualized human bodies. See also Le Guin (2002, 2006). For a useful summary and critique of recent musicological work on embodiment, see Maus (2010).

general, our knowledge of music is also embodied: we make sense of music—we understand it—according to patterns of bodily perception, activity, and feeling (Johnson 1997–98, 95).

When we understand one thing in terms of another, such as when we understand abstract concepts in terms of our bodily experience, we must employ metaphor. Traditionally, metaphor has usually been understood as a kind of linguistic flourish, a surface embellishment of language, with no deeper cognitive significance. Lakoff and Johnson (1980) argue, in contrast, that metaphor is the inescapable means by which we map knowledge across the domains of physical embodiment and abstract conceptualization:

> Metaphor pervades our normal conceptual system. Because so many of the concepts that are important to us are either abstract or not clearly delineated in our experience (the emotions, ideas, time, etc.), we need to get a grasp on them by means of other concepts that we understand in clearer terms (spatial orientations, objects, etc.). This need leads to metaphorical definition in our conceptual system (115).

Lakoff and Johnson have argued that metaphors tend to cluster into a relatively small number of "image-schemas," such as CONTAINERS, PATHS, LINKS, FORCES, BALANCE, UP-DOWN, FRONT-BACK, PART-WHOLE, CENTER-PERIPHERY (Lakoff 1987, 267).[6] Image-schemas are

> recurring, flexible patterns of our embodied interactions with our environments. They are the result of both the way we are structured physically as embodied organisms and the structure of our environments that permits only certain kinds of interactions with those environments. Moreover, they are not fixed templates that we impose on experience, but are instead highly flexible cross-modal patterns that make it possible for us to have ordered experiences that we can make some sense of. Image schemas like compulsive force, source-path-goal, balance, iteration, linkage, containment, and verticality are essential to our ability to have any meaningful experience at all, since they give us recurrent patterns and structured processes that we need to survive and flourish in our world (Johnson 1997–98, 97).

Many of the image-schemas described by Lakoff and Johnson have seemed suggestive to music theorists, including particularly CONTAINER, CYCLE, VERTICALITY, BALANCE, CENTER-PERIPHERY, FORCES, and SOURCE-PATH-GOAL. Recent work has identified these schemas both in standard music theories as well as in the melodic, harmonic, and formal organization of music.

Lakoff, Johnson, and other experientialists generally assume that everyone inhabits the same sort of normatively abled body. Thus, their work depends on what

---

6. In the experientialist literature, image-schemas are typically written in capital letters, a usage I follow here.

Garland-Thomson (2009, 45) calls "the phantom figure of the *normate*": "This neologism names the veiled subject position of the cultural self, the figure outlined by the array of deviant others whose marked bodies shore up the normate's boundaries" (Garland-Thomson 1997, 8). The normate body imagined by Lakoff and Johnson is a fiction, a phantom, an idealization, as opposed to the actual, concrete, and often disabled bodies that people really inhabit. Indeed, all of us, the normatively abled as well as the disabled, have experiences of disability and of the threat of disability.

Disability and the threat of disability are central to our experience of our bodies and are implicated in our conceptual image-schemas to a degree far beyond anything acknowledged by Lakoff and Johnson. We learn to experience BALANCE in moments when it is threatened or overturned by IMBALANCE. We can never experience BALANCE directly; rather, it is always experienced in relation to its opposing term. Likewise, we experience SOURCE-PATH-GOAL only in relation to the experience of BLOCKAGE, and we experience our bodies as a CONTAINER only when that container is PUNCTURED in some way (by the extrusion of something from inside the container or a wound from without) or its shape is DISTORTED (i.e., either expanded or compressed). In short, we know our abilities in relationship to our disabilities.[7] As a result, conceptualizations of music, depending as they must on bodily experience and embodied metaphors, are often shaped by disability. Although experientialists and music theorists have not acknowledged this, disability is among the bodily experiences that music and discourse about music may be understood to encode.

The remainder of this chapter is an attempt to explore that knowledge, to emphasize the ways in which disability has inflected the conceptualization of at least some music and at least some of our discourse about music. I will trace the role of particular image-schemas, including both the normative and nonnormative bodily states involved, in shaping discourse about music within three theoretical traditions. First, I will discuss the image-schema of the CONTAINER within studies of musical form. This critical tradition, which dates back to the beginning of the nineteenth century and has been reinvigorated by a series of highly visible and influential recent studies, is essentially concerned with the relationship of parts-to-whole and whole-to-parts in musical works, and with classifying musical works according to established formal types. I will show that theorists within that tradition often conceive of musical forms as containers, and do so most vividly at moments when the containers are ruptured or distorted in some way. Like a human body, a musical work has a form, and this form may be "deformed." In this way, I hope to show that studies of musical form deeply engage questions of disability.

7. BLOCKAGE is actually an image-schema identified by Johnson, but IMBALANCE, PUNCTURE, and DISTORTION are my own invention. Experientialism has tended to ignore the nonnormative, disabled counterparts of the bodily states and functions that underpin its image-schemas.

Second, I will discuss the image-schema of SOURCE-PATH-GOAL in the writings of Heinrich Schenker. Schenker's approach to the music of the eighteenth- and nineteenth-century canon remains dominant today in the English-speaking world, and has spawned a vast secondary literature devoted to refining and extending the analytical method and applying it to a larger corpus of musical works. Schenker is particularly concerned about the ways in which musical motion is enabled and the kinds of musical events that impede motion or, in extreme cases, paralyze the motion altogether

Third, I will discuss the image-schema of BALANCE in the writings of David Lewin. Lewin's "transformational theory" is the most significant development in music theory in the past several decades. In mathematically based studies of a variety of musical repertoires, Lewin shifts attention from the familiar objects of musical study (e.g., intervals, chords, melodies, keys) to the processes by which one object moves to another or is transformed into another.[8] In his own work and in that of his followers, Lewin's "transformational attitude" is frequently focused on inversional symmetry and balance. Rather than imagining symmetry as a static property that a particular chord might possess, Lewin thinks of it as a dynamic process that might lead the music from place to place. BALANCE and IMBALANCE are forces that act on music.

In all three theoretical traditions, disability (both its physical reality and the anxiety it induces) shapes the discourse. The nineteenth-century conception of the disabled body as something not unnatural but rather abnormal penetrates deeply into verbal descriptions of music.[9]

8. Here is Lewin's (1987, 158–59) own distillation of his transformational approach:

> To some extent for cultural-historical reasons, it is easier for us to hear "intervals" between individual objects than to hear transpositional relations between them; we are more used to conceiving transpositions as affecting Gestalts built up from individual objects. As this way of talking suggests, we are very much under the influence of Cartesian thinking in such matters. We tend to conceive the primary objects in our musical spaces as atomic individual "elements."... And we tend to imagine ourselves in the position of *observers* when we theorize about musical space; the space is "out there," away from our dancing bodies or singing voices.... In contrast, the transformational attitude is much less Cartesian. Given locations s and t in our space, this attitude does not ask for some observed measure of extension between reified "points"; rather it asks: "If I am *at* s and wish to get to t, what characteristic gesture should I perform in order to arrive there?"

9. The music theories I focus on here are mostly concerned with pitch. But theories of rhythm in the eighteenth and nineteenth centuries follow a similar logic. The relevant discussion has centered on the lengths of musical phrases, specifically how to explain the existence of odd or irregular phrase lengths in a musical world in which phrases of two, four, eight, and sixteen measures are so much more prevalent. Very roughly speaking, eighteenth-century theorists (e.g., Riepel, Kirnberger, and Koch) believed that duple phrase lengths are to be preferred as "the most natural," whereas nineteenth- and early twentieth-century theorists (e.g., Riemann and Prout) consider nonduple phrase lengths abnormal. As Rothstein (1989, 33) (the source for this discussion) has argued:

THEORIES OF FORM: ABNORMALITIES AND DEFORMATIONS

There are two persistent strains in studies of musical form that began at the end of the eighteenth century and became increasingly pronounced over the course of the nineteenth. The first is the conception of musical form as a CONTAINER, an arrangement of bounded spaces that contain musical content (themes or harmonies). FORM IS A CONTAINER is an embodied image-schema. Through it we understand that musical form can speak to us of human bodies, and that musical forms, like human bodies, may be *well formed* or *deformed*. The possibility of *formal deformation* links this conception of musical form to the history of disability.

A second strain in form studies is the sense that form is a norm—a normative or conventional arrangement of musical elements. In this sense, forms may be *normal* or *abnormal*. FORM IS A NORM is not an embodied image-schema, but the possibility of *formal abnormality* links this conception also to the history of disability.

These two strains in the history of form studies are closely intertwined—musical form may be understood as a conventional mold, that is, a normative container.[10] In form studies, the sense of form as a normative container (an approach that Mark Evan Bonds calls "conformational") coexists with a diametrically opposed sense of form as the unique shape of an individual work (an approach that Bonds calls "generative").[11] The generative approach held the aesthetic and moral high ground

---

> Authors such as Riemann and Prout have held that *all* phrases of non-duple length—those of other than two, four, eight, or sixteen measures—can best be understood as variations of "normal" phrases of duple length. Riemann goes so far as to warn composers that they can never escape the norm of the eight-measure period, even if they try, any more than they can escape the laws of tonality.... Gradually, asymmetrical phrases—especially those of odd-numbered lengths—came to be looked upon with something resembling moral disapproval.

My thanks to Scott Murphy for calling my attention to rhythmic theory as a normalizing enterprise.

10. As Newman (1983, 110) contends,

> Form may be viewed, textbook fashion, as a *mold* or standardized design, with all the conveniences of quick reference that such classifications permit and all the dangers of Procrustean analysis and false criteria that they pose. Approaching a form as a mold puts the emphasis on everything that is typical or common practice, if not commonplace. Our best illustration, of course, is textbook "sonata form," itself.

11. Bonds (1991, 13–14) writes:

> The concept of musical form encompasses two basic perspectives that differ radically from each other. On the one hand, "form" is often used to denote those various structural elements that a large number of works share in common. In terms of practical analysis, this approach to form looks for lowest common denominators and views individual works in comparison with such stereotypical patterns as sonata form, rondo, ABA, and the like. For the sake of convenience, this view of form may be called "conformational," as it is based on the comparison of a specific work against an abstract, ideal type. The contrasting perspective sees form as the unique shape of a specific work. This view, unlike the first, is essentially generative, in that it considers how each individual work grows from within and how the various elements of a work coordinate to make a coherent whole. In its most extreme manifestations, the generative idea of form makes no essential distinction between the form and content of a given work.

through much of the twentieth century. Indeed, it is hard to find a study of musical form from the twentieth century that does not contain a denunciation of taxonomies, "jelly-moulds" (Tovey), or stereotypical patterns.[12] But even the most ardent generativists have found it hard to escape entirely the image-schemas of containers and norms; these have proven remarkably persistent, and not only in the textbooks. Furthermore, the three most important contemporary studies of form—those of Bonds,[13] Caplin,[14] and Hepokoski and Darcy[15]—have all taken approaches that are explicitly conformational, at least in some degree.

12. Tovey (1949a, 289): "The art forms of Haydn, Mozart, and Beethoven were not moulds in which music could be cast, but inner principles by which the music grew." Richard Strauss made the same point somewhat more colorfully in a 1888 letter to Bulow, cited in Newman (1983, 35–36):

> Now, what was for Beethoven a "form" absolutely in congruity with the highest, most glorious content, is now, after 60 years, used as a formula inseparable from our instrumental music (which I strongly dispute), simply to accommodate and enclose a "pure musical" (in the strictest and narrowest meaning of the word) content, or worse, to stuff and expand a content with which it does not correspond.... We cannot have any more random patterns, that mean nothing either to the composer or the listener, and no symphonies (Brahms excepted, of course) that always give me the impression of being giant's clothes, made to fit a Hercules, in which a thin tailor is trying to comport himself elegantly.

More recently, see Webster (2001, 688): "Sonata form is not a mould into which the composer has poured the contents...each movement grows bar by bar and phrase by phrase, with the meaning of each event depending both on its function in the structure and its dramatic context."

13. Bonds (1991, 14, 29) writes:

> Both [generative and conformational] approaches are valid, yet neither is sufficient for musical analysis. Looking for stereotypical patterns can help call attention to deviations from a recognized norm, but it cannot explain these deviations. At the same time, analyzing a work entirely "from within" cannot account for the striking structural similarities that exist among a large number of quite independent works.... What is needed, then, is a general theory of form that can account for conventional patterns and at the same time do justice to the immense diversity that exists within the framework of these patterns.

14. Caplin (1998, 4) writes:

> The theory [set forth in this book] establishes strict formal categories but applies them flexibly in analysis. One reason that the traditional *Formenlehre* has fallen out of favor with many historians and theorists is their belief that the use of rigid, abstract categories of form results too often in Procrustean analyses that obscure diversities in style and distort the individuality of the musical work. Yet forsaking categories would make it almost impossible to generalize about formal organization, and such a situation runs counter to most musicians' intuitions that classical form features regularly recurring patterns of conventionalized procedures.

15. Hepokoski and Darcy (1997, 116–17) write:

> In our view, moment-to-moment compositional choices may be profitably understood as elements of an ongoing dialogue with reasonably ascertainable, flexible generic norms.... Our aim has been twofold: first, to (re-)generate those norms—again, inductively (under the conviction that the most valuable treatises on late-eighteenth-century "sonata form" were written by the great masters, not by the early theorists); second, to configure the norms into an ordered description of standard practices, deformations, and overrides that we call "Sonata Theory" (with capital S and capital T).

Bonds' "frameworks" and Caplin's "categories" are both kinds of containers—formal spaces that can be filled by various kinds of musical content. More obviously and explicitly, so are Hepokoski and Darcy's "zones" and "spaces."[16] Intrinsic to the image-schema of the CONTAINER is the possibility that the container can be ruptured or distorted. Indeed, the sense of a formal unit as a container is perhaps most strongly felt just at the moments when the its exterior shell is breached, or when the container is suddenly forced to change shape under pressure from its internal contents. Caplin's terms for this phenomenon are *elision, evasion, deception,* and *falseness* (as in a "false recapitulation"), suggesting transgression of a boundary that is not only formal but possibly moral as well. Hepokoski and Darcy's (1997, 131) even more suggestive term is *deformation,* defined as "a strikingly unusual or strained procedure relying on our knowledge of the typical limits of the norm." If musical form can be understood metaphorically as a human body via the image-schema of the container, then deformations in musical form may metaphorically suggest deformations in a human body. Hepokoski and Darcy's use of the term "deformation" simply makes explicit what is already implicit in any conformational theory of musical form: a musical form, understood as a normative container, is a metaphorical human body, and thus formal deformations can be understood as bodily disfigurements.[17]

Their "Sonata Theory" is given its fullest exposition in Hepokoski and Darcy (2006). The central role of norms and deformations is evident from the title of that book. See also Hepokoski (2001–2002, 2002). It would not be accurate to describe the Sonata Theory of Hepokoski and Darcy as strictly conformational:

Sonata Theory starts from the premise that an individual composition is a musical utterance that is set (by the composer) into a dialogue with implied norms. This is an understanding of formal procedures as *dynamic, dialogic.* As such our conception of the sonata as an instance of *dialogic form* is not accurately described as seeking to reinstate a bluntly 'conformational' view of that structure (Hepokoski and Darcy 2006, 10).

But at the very least, like Bonds's "patterns" and Caplin's "categories," the "norms" of Hepokoski and Darcy create a template against which to understand deviations and deformations.

16. As Hepokoski and Darcy (2006, 16) describe their zones and spaces,

The normative sonata consists of three musical spaces (again, the exposition, development, and recapitulation).... Each of the three spaces is usually subjected to thematic and textural differentiation. Each is marked by several successive themes and textures, all of which are normally recognizable as generically appropriate for their specified location.

The authors argue that their spaces and zones should not be understood as mere inert containers to be filled but rather as "complex sets (or constellations) of flexible action-options devised to facilitate the dialogue [with a backdrop of implied norms]" (11). However, any spatial model of form engages the image-schema of the container in some way. By their very nature, spaces are bounded, with an exterior and an interior, separated by a boundary or shell, and the interior space is available to be filled.

17. The suggestiveness of the term *deformation* takes us beyond the meaning explicitly attached to it by Hepokoski and Darcy (2006), who assert that it need carry no connotation of actual human disability:

While we do intend "deformation" to imply a strain and distortion of the norm—the composer's application of uncommon creative force toward the production of a singular

It is paradox worth pondering that deformities are valued so differently in life and in art. Formal deviations, which are dealt with harshly in real life when manifested as bodily deformities, may be prized within art, and sonatas with "deformations" are often the most interesting and expressive ones.[18] Here is an area in which music may have a singular contribution to make to Disability Studies. In literary forms, disabled characters are generally stigmatized and disposed of after playing their crucial role of setting the drama in motion; in musical forms, the "deformations" are often the most highly valued.[19] Either way, however, conformational theories of musical form, and the musical forms themselves when viewed conformationally, may be understood to be metaphorically about normal and deviant bodies, and thus to participate in the construction of the culture and history of disability.

As a central canon of acknowledged musical masterworks began to coalesce in the middle of the nineteenth century (far later in music than in the other arts), musicians began studying and talking about musical form in systematic ways. That involved a significant reorientation in conceptions of musical form, roughly speaking from one that views musical forms as ideal types, to be used as models for emulation by composers, to one that views them in terms of statistical norms, to be used as objects for analysis and contemplation.[20] The focus of the inquiry into musical form, like the simultaneous inquiry into the meaning of disability, shifted from what is ideal or natural to what is statistically normal.

---

aesthetic effect—we do not use this term in its looser, more colloquial sense, one that can connote a negative sense of aesthetic defectiveness, imperfection, or ugliness.... Within our system, "deformation" is only a technical term referring to a striking way of stretching or overriding a norm (614–15).

Clearly the term *deformation* can be used in something like a neutral manner to suggest simply "alteration of form or shape." But that sense is only the third of the definitions listed in the *Oxford English Dictionary*. The first two are "The action (or result) of deforming or marring the form or beauty of; disfigurement, defacement" and "Alteration of form for the worse." The neutral, nonevaluative usage cannot fully escape the historical resonance of the more familiar use of the term.

18. The differential treatment of disability in art and in life is a familiar theme in the Disability Studies literature:

While disability's troubling presence provides literary works with the potency of an unsettling cultural commentary, disabled people have been historically refused a parallel power with their social institutions. In other words, while literature often relies on disability's transgressive potential, disabled people have been sequestered, excluded, exploited, and obliterated on the very basis of which their literary representation so often rests. Literature serves up disability as a repressed deviation from cultural imperatives of normativity, while disabled populations suffer the consequences of representational association with deviance and recalcitrant corporeal difference. The paradox of these two deployments, artistic versus historical, cannot be reconciled (Mitchell and Snyder 2000, 8–9).

19. This contrast between literature and music in their stigmatization or valorization of disabled characters comes from Bruce Quaglia (private communication).

20. According to Burnham (2002, 800), the analysis of large-scale tonal form became

By the end of the nineteenth century, the study of musical form had taken a decisive empirical turn, one that has endured until the present, although under continual critique (in some cases by the empiricists themselves).[21] It is assumed by Prout and Tovey, as it is more recently by Blume, Newman, and Hepokoski and Darcy, that the study of musical form involves the inspection of lots of pieces and their categorization based on shared attributes, which is implicitly a process of statistical norming in which most of the population is sheltered under the bell-shaped curve, with abnormal members relegated to the margins.[22] The

---

a central preoccupation of music-theoretical writings ever since the "work concept" (consolidated around 1800) decisively shifted theoretical focus to whole works of music and thus to overall form. The analysis of musical forms began in this context as a pedagogical exercise in emulation....But by the end of the nineteenth century, the business of formal analysis began to be undertaken as a kind of research program—what was primarily at stake was no longer the education of a young composer but rather the viability of theories of music that attempted to determine what were felt to be the natural laws of music. Pedagogy gave way to taxonomy, emulation to contemplation.

21. Prout (1895, iii) gives a personal and evocative account of this implicitly statistical methodology:

In the preface to *Musical Form* [an earlier work by Prout] it was said that that work had involved more labour than any of its predecessors. But the compilation of that volume proved to be mere child's play in comparison with the research necessary for the present one, which has required more than eighteen months' hard work to complete it. This has been the inevitable result of the system on which the author has worked. Though he has consulted numerous theoretical treatises, he has in no case taken either his statements or his illustrations at second hand; in every single instance he has gone direct to the works of the great masters, both for his rules and for his examples. What this involves may be judged from one or two illustrations. Before writing the three paragraphs on the Minuet, the author examined every minuet in the complete works of Handel, Bach, Couperin, Corelli, Mozart, Beethoven, and Schubert, the whole of Haydn's 83 quartets, all the symphonies (about fifty) which he possesses by the same composer, and a number of miscellaneous specimens by other writers. The result of all this work occupies less than three pages. Even more laborious were the preliminary investigations for the sonata form. About 1,200 movements were carefully examined before a line of the text was written; and this task occupied the whole of the author's spare time for nearly a month.

Apparently Prout studied roughly forty movements per day during his "spare time." A similar empirical approach characterizes the Sonata Theory of Hepokoski and Darcy, which is

...generated inductively from the analysis of hundreds of sonatas, symphonies, overtures, quartets, and other chamber music from the late eighteenth- and early nineteenth-century repertory. The works examined include not only those of Haydn, Mozart, and Beethoven, but also those of other composer preceding and surrounding them, including Sammartini, Stamitz, Cannabich, J. C. Bach, C. P. E. Bach, Dittersdorf, Boccherini, Clementi, Dussek, Cherubini, and others (Hepokoski and Darcy 1997, 116).

22. This new orientation toward statistical norming is described and critiqued in Rosen (1972, 32):

The most dangerous aspect of the traditional theory of "sonata form" is the normative one....The assumption that divergences from the pattern are irregularities is made as often as the inference that earlier eighteenth-century versions of the form represent an inferior stage from which a higher type evolved. This is implied, too, but in a more specious way, in a good deal of twentieth-century musical thought. Now the attitude is

conformational wing of the *Formenlehre* (Form Studies) tradition, with its implicitly statistical methodology and its insistence on distinguishing the normal from the abnormal, teaches us what it means for a musical form to conform to or transgress conventional norms and therefore also may assist in teaching us what it means to have a normative or nonnormative body.

The rich *Formenlehre* tradition, including its recent efflorescence in the work of Bonds, Caplin, and Hepokoski and Darcy, has depended from the beginning on what has come to seem a self-evident concept of the normal, understood fundamentally as a statistical norm.[23] The idea that a body (or anything else) can be normal or abnormal seems perfectly natural and self-evident, but it is an idea with a history bound up with the history of disability. In fact, the concepts of normal and abnormal emerge in a particular time and place—Western Europe in roughly the first half of the nineteenth century—partly as a response to changes in the cultural construction of disability and the material circumstances of people with disabilities.[24]

Prior to roughly 1840, the relevant constellation of words (i.e., normal, normalcy, normality, norm, abnormal) had not existed in any European language.[25]

---

statistical rather than hortative: the pattern for "sonata form" is no longer an idealized one but is based on the common practice of eighteenth-century composers. "Sonata form" is taken to mean the form generally used by a majority of composers at a given time.

The "statistical attitude" is apparent in Blume (1979) and Newman (1983).

23. The more recent form studies may err in conflating the normative with the statistically most common. The normative need not be especially common to establish a regulating standard against with others are constructed is deviants. Extending metaphorically from musical bodies to human bodies, I observe that the normative body is white, male, straight, nondisabled, but those bodies actually comprise a small minority of human bodies.

24. The following discussion is based on Davis (1995), particularly chapter 2, "Constructing Normalcy." See also Branson and Miller (2002, 37–38):

[In the early nineteenth century], the concept of normality entered not only the language of science but also the language of everyday life, especially that of the middle classes for whom the distinction between normality and pathology became a vital source of social control.... The concept of normality remained and remains at all times insecure, dependent on its opposite and in constant need of reaffirmation. A view of a diverse humanity that was imbued with almost infinite difference gave way to a view of an essentially uniform humanity that was surrounded on its edges, on its margins, by the pathological foils to that uniformity or "normality." But no "pathological" population could exist until one was culturally constructed.

25. In English (according to the *Oxford English Dictionary*), the word "normal" (in its original sense of "standing at right angles") dates back to the seventeenth century, with roots in Latin, but in its modern sense of "constituting, conforming to, not deviating or differing from, the common type of standard; regular, usual," its earliest use is given as 1828, and it only becomes common after around 1840. In French, the first appearance of the adjective "normal" or "normale" in the *Dictionnaire de L'Académie française* comes in the Sixth Edition (1832–35). According to the *Deutches Wörterbuch von Jacob Grimm und Wilhelm Grimm*, the first use of the term "normal" in German in its modern sense dates from the mid-1850s. Of course, there may be a significant lapse of time between the emergence of a concept and the emergence of terms used to express it. Certainly a kind of casual statistical norming

The middle of the nineteenth century witnessed the emergence of the science of statistics and the associated practice of studying populations and evaluating them in relation to particular traits, such as intelligence or height. From the beginning, the practice of statistical norming, in which most people are located under a bell-shaped curve with the rest relegated to its margins, was associated with eugenics, a desire to purge society of people defined as abnormal or deviant.[26] At the historical moment when people with disabilities began to emerge as a distinctive class, with a new set of institutions to educate, train, and treat them, statistics and eugenics also emerged, with their concepts of normal and abnormal, to contain and marginalize the disabled.[27]

But the very usefulness of the statistical norm has tended, ironically, to normalize and naturalize the concept itself and to obscure its history, which is closely linked to changing conceptualizations of the human body and, in particular, the disabled human body. Both the normal musical form and the normal human body are cultural constructions of a particular time and place. Restoring our sense of their intertwined histories enriches our understanding of both.

SCHENKER'S THEORY OF HARMONY AND VOICE LEADING: NORMALIZATION AND PARALYSIS

For Heinrich Schenker, steeped in the organicist tradition, a musical work is a human body and thus subject to forces that threaten to disable it. For him, the organic nature of a composition, its living body, is exemplified in the relationship among its structural levels:

(e.g., "that guy over there doesn't look like the rest of us") is presumably a pretty common and long-standing notion. What is new in the mid-nineteenth century is the conceptualization of the normal in implicitly or explicitly statistical terms, as something that situates individuals in relation to large populations with respect to particular traits.

26. The career of Francis Galton may be taken as emblematic of the intertwining of the history of statistics (with its foundational interest in sorting populations into normal and abnormal) and the history of eugenics (with its foundational interest in purging society of people with disabilities). Galton was both a pioneering figure in statistics (the originator of concepts like "regression" and the "correlation coefficient") and a founder of a political movement for eugenics, a term he coined. See Brookes (2004).

27. Davis (1995, 29–30) writes:

The concept of a norm, unlike that of an ideal, implies that the majority of the population must or should somehow be part of the norm. The norm pins down that majority of the population that falls under the arch of the standard bell-shaped curve.... With the concept of the norm comes the concept of deviations or extremes. When we think of bodies, in a society where the concept of the norm is operative, then people with disabilities will be thought of as deviants.... Statistics is bound up with eugenics because the central insight of statistics is the idea that a population can be normed. An important consequence of the idea of the norm is that it divides the total population into standard and nonstandard subpopulations. The next step in conceiving of the population as norm and non-norm is for the state to attempt to norm the nonstandard—the aim of eugenics.

Musical coherence can be achieved only through the fundamental structure in the background and its transformations in the middleground and foreground. It should have been evident long ago that the same principle applies both to a musical organism and to the human body: it grows outward from within. Therefore it would be fruitless as well as incorrect to attempt to draw conclusions about the organism from its epidermis. The hand, legs, and ears of the human body do not begin to grow after birth; they are present at the time of birth. Similarly, in a composition, a limb which was not somehow born with the middle and background cannot grow to be a diminution (Schenker 1979, 6).[28]

Whereas Schoenberg was concerned with a work confronting its "tonal problem" as it unfolds in time, Schenker was more concerned about the drama of the relationship among the structural levels. There, too, elements may occur at the later levels (the levels nearer the musical surface) that it is the business of the earlier levels to neutralize, absorb, and "normalize."[29] Schenkerian analytical practice, for both pitch and rhythm, always involves normalization—musical events are understood in relationship to the normative prototypes they transform or displace.[30] The analytical process involves normalizing the abnormal. This way of approaching music, however familiar it may be, is not inevitable or natural, but historically contingent, and involves the intertwining of the history of music theory with the history of disability.

28. Schenker similarly observed that,

> Just as man, animal and plant are configurations sprung from the smallest seed—perhaps the stars are also configurations from substantially simpler entities—so also are all compositions by geniuses configurations born of only a few intervals, which can be clearly identified through the perspective of the voice-leading strata (Schenker 1996, 18).

29. "Normalization" is a term that originates with William Rothstein. Rothstein applies the term primarily to tonal rhythm—he shows that a variety of surface rhythms can be understood as displacements of an underlying norm—but he describes the concept in terms sufficiently general as to embrace pitch as well:

> In tonal music we continually hear the specific, the distinctive, and the surprising in relation to the general, the normal, and the expected; *the abnormal is understood in terms of the normal* [emphasis added]. Tension is understood to arise from the difference between the given musical phenomena (which, in a piece of any artistic interest, are bound to contain surprises and abnormalities) and the musical norms from which those phenomena depart. The distance between the musical surface and the underlying norms fluctuates within a composition, yielding for the listener a corresponding fluctuation of tension (Rothstein 1990, 89).

Technically, Rothstein uses the term to describe realignments of notes between the musical surface and a voice-leading reduction, or between two levels of a voice-leading reduction, with the process of normalization applied anew at each successive level of reduction.

30. This attitude underpins every theory of tonal harmony post-1850, and is particularly conspicuous in the pedagogy of tonal harmony. Students are taught what is normative and warned away from the abnormal. It is in that spirit that Aldwell and Schachter (1989, 319) describe weak-beat cadential 6/4 chords as "deviant."

In this underlying dialectic of normal and abnormal, Schenker's musical thought reflects the same historical and cultural forces as those that shape the tradition of form studies. In both cases, a large population of musical works is normed with respect to certain desirable traits, with anomalous events understood as abnormal. Furthermore, in both cases, the normative takes on a coercive force: the abnormal must be normalized (or, at least, rationalized with respect to the norm). By engaging the dichotomy of normal and abnormal, Schenker's theory both reflects and participates in the history and cultural construction of disability.

For Schenker, the principal musical abnormality requiring normalization is dissonance. Dissonance, if properly contained within what he called a "linear progression," is a principal source of musical content, interest, and motion (a linear progression is a stepwise structural line that guides the music). But if dissonances are allowed to pile up outside the control of the linear progressions, the musical body becomes disabled. Properly controlled, dissonance enables mobility; uncontrolled, dissonances impair mobility—they produce musical "paralysis," as Schenker demonstrated in a series of highly critical discussions of Rameau, Riemann, Schoenberg, and Stravinsky.

In viewing dissonance in this way, Schenker participated in a long tradition in Western music theory of regarding dissonance as something potentially threatening to the consonant framework that simultaneously constrains it and gives it meaning (Cohen 1993). Dissonance is needed (for expressive purposes, and to propel the music forward), but simultaneously stigmatized as undesirable and threatening to the integrity of the structure. For Schenker, as for many other theorists, consonance is associated with the normative, healthy body and dissonance with the possibility of abnormality, deformation, and paralysis.

Schenker's understanding of the effects of dissonance was embodied, drawing on the bodily image-schema of SOURCE-PATH-GOAL and the associated schema of BLOCKAGE. For Schenker the linear progression is the principal source of musical continuity and coherence and it has the metaphorical trajectory of a body in motion from a source, along a path, toward a goal: "Every linear progression shows the eternal shape of life—birth to death. The linear progression begins, lives its own existence in the passing tones, ceases when it has reached its goal—all as organic as life itself" (Schenker 1979, 44). In the course of its journey from source to goal, the musical body may encounter obstacles that threaten to impede the motion. In most cases, such blockages are a vital part of the music, creating interest and content. Without them, a musical work would be boring and extremely short— the eventual attainment of the concluding tonic would represent no significant achievement at all: "In the art of music, as in life, motion toward the goal encounters obstacles, reverses, disappointments, and involves great distances, detours, expansions, interpolations, and, in short, retardations or all kinds" (Schenker 1979, 5). Like Schoenberg's tonal problems, and like Hepokoski and Darcy's sonata deformations, Schenker's blockages suggest the aesthetic value of disability, a value that is enshrined in a great deal of art of all kinds. Often, it seems, the works we value most are those that deal in some way with the threat or reality of disability. Usually, such works successfully contain the disability, but it must be vigorously present in order to be satisfyingly contained.

Blockages may be aesthetically desirable if they generate interest and content, but if they cannot be dislodged, then the motion stops and the music becomes paralyzed. For Schenker, the most troubling kind of blockage results from an excess of VERTICALITY, another embodied image-schema. Instead of flowing forward along normative linear pathways, the notes may be piled up in vertical stacks, fatally arresting the sense of motion along a path toward a goal. It is precisely that excess of verticality, and the resulting musical paralysis, that Schenker criticized in a chorale setting by Hugo Riemann: "The setting [of a chorale melody] by Hugo Riemann illustrates the latter-day disastrous growth of chords in the exclusively vertical sense. These 'chords' paralyze [Ger. *unterbinden*] the contrapuntal flow of the bass as well as that of the inner voices" (Schenker 1979, 96). In their autonomous verticality, Riemann's chords inhibit the contrapuntal flow. Riemann's bass line, in particular, is a disjunct series of chordal roots rather than the kind of melodic line that might have formed itself into linear progressions.

The disabling paralysis that afflicts Riemann's chorale setting can be traced to the musical theories of Rameau, as seen in the title of Schenker's essay "Rameau or Beethoven? Creeping Paralysis or Spiritual Potency in Music?" (Schenker 1997).[31] Musical paralysis results when composers fail to compose "with the sensually vital motion of [music's] innate horizontal linear progressions, patterns that correspond with the motions of the human soul" and focus instead on vertical harmonic combinations (Schenker 1997, 4). Schenker blamed Rameau for the resulting paralysis:

> In Rameau's fundamental idea there lurked an element of the mechanical—turned away from the living art of voice-leading—right from the start, but that first mechanical element engendered mechanism upon mechanism in its train. Little by little, the seventh, whether as passing note or suspension, and the ninth, whether as suspension or changing-note, were made out to be chord-components, from which it was but a short step to bona fide seventh and ninth chords. Once on this slippery slope, nothing could stop recognition being given also to eleventh and thirteenth chords; and so, today, things have reached such a pass that, on pretext of the higher partials of the overtone series, any and every piling-up of notes, no matter how it may have come about, is indiscriminately taken for a chord. Make no mistake: Rameau's error has been compounded

31. The German word that Bent translates as "paralysis" is *Erstarrung*. Bent (in Schenker 1997, 1) comments:

> Schenker's motivic use of *Erstarrung* and *erstarren* throughout the first two-thirds of this essay presents the translator with a conundrum, for the verb *erstarren* has a range of meanings, from "stiffen," through "congeal," "coagulate," "solidify," "freeze," to "become numb," "torpid," "paralyzed," and Schenker exploits this range such that no one English word will work idiomatically.

to the limit, the followers of Rameau's theory have reached a point of no return. Paralysis! (Schenker 1997, 5).[32]

Although Schenker blamed Rameau, the real villains are those contemporary composers who pile up notes into complex, dissonant harmonies. If a work of music is metaphorically a body, then an excess of verticality, particularly if it involves the piling up of dissonant notes, is a disabling condition, one that restricts and potentially paralyzes movement. The dissonances, instead of creating motion under the control of a linear progression, impede the motion—they are a fatally disabling obstacle on the path traversed by the musical body.

It is just this disabling condition that, for Schenker, characterizes the modern music of his time. Once the dissonances have liberated themselves from the control of the linear progressions, once they are "emancipated," in Schoenberg's term, the result, according to Schenker, is theoretical confusion and musical paralysis, as in Stravinsky's Piano Concerto:

> A setting like Stravinsky's is insufficient even for certifying dissonances, because the only surety even for dissonances—and this is the crux of the matter—is the cohesiveness of a well-organized linear progression: without cohesiveness, dissonances do not even exist! Thus it is completely futile when Stravinsky imagines that he can make the dissonance still more dissonant by piling up dissonances (or, to put in the language of Schoenberg, who equates dissonance with consonance, make the consonance more consonant). It is futile to masquerade all the inability to create tension by means of appropriate linear progressions as freedom, and to proclaim that nothing bad exists in music at all (Schenker 1996, 18).

The "piling up of dissonances" thus impairs the mobility of the linear progressions. Such dissonances are beyond the recuperative power of normalization.

Fictional characters with disabilities tend to conform to a small number of "cultural scripts." It appears that when musical works are conceived of in terms of disability, they also enact familiar stereotypes. As noted earlier, the first movement of Beethoven's Third Symphony is a Heroic Overcomer, who triumphs blazingly over the potentially disabling C-sharp of its opening; the Finale of his Eighth Symphony

---

32. In referring to the higher partials of the overtone series as a justification for complex harmonies, Schenker seems to have Schoenberg in mind, in particular a passage from Schoenberg's *Theory of Harmony* (Schoenberg 1978, 21):

> The expressions "consonance" and "dissonance," which signify an antithesis, are false. It all simply depends on the growing ability of the analyzing ear to familiarize itself with the remote overtones, thereby expanding the conception of what is euphonious, suitable for art, so that it embraces the whole natural phenomenon. What today is remote can tomorrow be close at hand; it is all a matter of whether one can get closer. And the evolution of music has followed this course: it has drawn into the stock of artistic resources more and more of the harmonic possibilities inherent in the tone.

is a Comic Misadventurer, whose stumbles are a source of crude humor; and Schubert's Moment Musical is a Saintly Sage, who achieves an otherworldly wisdom through the experience of disability. In the same sense, Stravinsky's Piano Concerto, in Schenker's view, is an Obsessive Avenger whose piling up of dissonances outside the control of linear progressions threatens to lay waste to traditional tonality.[33]

Schenker's quoted comments are in reference to a particular work of Stravinsky's—his Piano Concerto—but are obviously applicable to an entire repertoire that Schenker detested. Schenker thus suggests that an entire repertoire can be disabled. A repertoire is also a body—a *corpus* of work. And like an individual piece, an entire body of work can become disabled through excessive verticality and unregulated dissonance. That, for Schenker, is the problem of atonality: it represents disability or abnormality with respect to well-formed, normal, "natural" tonality:

> Today it is the fashion to talk about an "excess of technique," an excess that allegedly stifles the composer. If we could only gain clarity about what this slogan really means! Is technique not the fulfillment on the part of the artist of those demands which the subject matter itself, far above the artist, imposes on him? In pursuit of such fulfillment, is not technique then a necessary, good, and—so to speak—healthy thing? Is not the technique of a work comparable to the health of a body whose organs fulfill all the functions nature demands of them? If we mean technique in its authentic and true significance, how can we speak logically of an "excess of technique"? Does anyone ever speak seriously of an excess of health? How could this be more than simply health itself? ... [Today's composers] try to make up for their shortcomings by stuffing their sounds with the excelsior of passing tones. Indeed, passing tones are the sum and substance of today's pompously flaunted technique. If composers could at least demonstrate a greater mastery of this art! But even here a secure instinct and reliable aural skills are lacking: inadvertently comical discords are generated instead of forthright conflicts between several voices. The present era, which is guilty of using this latest non-technique for the first time in the history of our art, was also the one to find a suitable name for it: generally it is called "cacophony" (Schenker 1987, xxi–xxii).

For Schenker, then, modern music as a whole is disabled and unhealthy, with its organs functioning improperly. Just as it is the business of each piece to heal its own wounds and normalize its own abnormalities, Schenker took as his historical task to cure music of the disability of atonality.[34]

For Schenker, the threat of disability, particularly paralysis, lurks both within individual works and within repertoires, and the awareness of this threat is fundamental

33. These disability stereotypes are all derived from the study of film in Norden 1996.
34. Schenker is not the only critic to pathologize atonal music as a disability, a monstrous perversion of nature—that has long been a commonplace—nor is atonal music the only

to his musical thinking. Within individual works by the masters of the tonal tradition, that threat can be contained by the normalizing power of the fundamental structure. For Schoenberg, the process of normalizing the abnormal unfolds diachronically: a tonal problem is introduced and, over the course of a piece, brought into conformity with normative tonality. For Schenker, the process unfolds synchronically, in the relationship among the structural levels: dissonances and their tendency toward excessive verticality are ultimately normalized within the fundamental structure. But, for Schenker, the threat posed by atonality to the body of common-practice tonal works is not so easily contained. Indeed, Schenker believed that music had been left permanently disabled (i.e., paralyzed) by the emancipation of the dissonance.

LEWIN'S TRANSFORMATIONAL THEORY: BALANCE AND SYMMETRY

An interest in inversional symmetry established, challenged, and possibly regained underpins a number of the more recent theoretical traditions that have accreted around Schoenberg and Webern's free atonal music, particularly the work of David Lewin. Lewin has consistently argued that inversion has the potential for inducing a sense of musical balance: one group of notes is symmetrically balanced against another around a central note (or notes). The resulting balance can be felt as an ideal, stable, harmonious state, explicitly analogous to the physical balance of the normal, nondisabled human body. The balance can be disrupted, and the disruption may set in motion a musical effort to restore the balance. Inversion is thus a process that can motivate musical movement.

Lewin derives these ideas in part from the music and theories of Schoenberg, as discussed in chapter 4. For Schoenberg, disruptions of balance often created "tonal problems"—disturbances in the musical flow, deviations from the norm, potentially disabling conditions that create a problem to be solved, or a defect for which a cure is sought. Lewin prefers instead metaphors of questioning, seeking, searching, and desiring.[35] Notes may be understood to search for their absent inversional partners, and such a search may be resolved, in the manner of a dissonance resolving to a consonance, when the absent partner appears.[36]

When two harmonies are nearly but not quite related by inversion, the music may convey an "urge" or a sense of "lust" toward symmetry and balance. As Lewin

---

repertoire to be pathologized in this way. According to Stras (2009, 300), jazz was treated in a similar manner by some of its early critics: "In the early twentieth century, jazz was condemned in explicitly pathological terms.... Clear associations between jazz and disability were expressed by sociologists, physicians, music critics and musicians, and were promulgated in both the specialist and popular press."

35. This theoretical framework, including the metaphors of search, resolution, urge, and lust, is employed in Lewin (1982–83). See also Lewin (1987, 1993, 1997).

36. Lewin's technical, analytical discussion of the opening of Webern's Movement for String Quartet, Op. 5, No 2, a work discussed in chapter 4, suggests the possibility of a note searching for its inversional partner:

says with respect to Schoenberg's Little Piano Piece, Op. 19, No. 6, "I find it suggestive to think of these generative lusts as musical tensions and/or potentialities
which later events of the piece will resolve and/or realize to greater or lesser extents"
(Lewin 1982–83, 341).

Lewin's analysis of Webern's Orchestra Pieces, Op. 10, Nos. 3 and 4, is likewise evocative of Lewin's theoretical interest in inversional balance and some of
the associated rhetoric of searching and desiring. Lewin observes that a high
C-sharp at the beginning of No. 3 "maximally discombobulates the symmetric
structure." Much of Lewin's analysis is a description of the music's attempts to
reestablish the symmetrical balance. I quote a bit of the analysis here not so much
for the musical specifics as for the suggestive rhetoric, mostly of implicit questions seeking answers:

> Since the pitch structure of the Shimmer sonority [first chord of No. 3] is almost sym-
> metrical by inversion about A_4, there is a certain urge for the high $C\#_6$ of the Shimmer
> to be "answered" by a low F_3. That does not happen [immediately, but] the next pitch
> class, after (about six seconds of) Shimmer, is an F, specifically the F_5 that begins the
> Tune. The C# is thus answered as a pitch class, if not as a pitch. The pitch F_3 does not
> appear in Op. 10, No. 3, but it does appear very audibly as the first "bass note" of Op. 10,
> No. 4, where it is coupled into a verticality beneath Db4. Perhaps the low $\{F_3, Db_4\}$ dyad
> at the opening of Op. 10, No. 4 answers by inversion-about-A_4 the high $C\#_6$ of Shimmer
> plus the F_5 of the Tune. That is quite conjectural. Much clearer is the desire of the
> Shimmer C# to find some F that answers it by pitch-class inversion-about-A. The F at
> the beginning of the Tune is one such F. An even stronger F appears at the reprise of the
> Shimmer sonority.... (Lewin 1993, 88).[37]

Under such circumstances, a state of imbalance may be experienced as a defect,
which the musical body may seek to recuperate. Indeed, the musical discourse of
certain pieces may be understood as a series of efforts to reestablish, or to create, a
sense of inversional balance and symmetry.

> In measure 1, the dyad (G, B) becomes extended to X = (G, B, C#) and the melody lin-
> gers on the high point C#. The questioning effect of this gesture is interrelated with a
> search in the music for E♭ = I(C#) and (A, F, E♭) = I(X), a search which is to some extent
> resolved by the chord of measure 2, where the C# and the X trichord that embeds it find
> their I-partners (Lewin 1982–83, 312).

37. Likewise, see Lewin (1997), which argues that the opening of the first song in Schoenberg's
Pierrot Lunaire involves "rival centers of inversion" that "throw the structure inherently off
balance." Later, the balance is restored, creating a sense of closure:

> In the pitch-class world, I_1 wants to balance with F#/G, or with C/C#; I_2 wants to
> balance "a semitone away" with G alone, or with C# alone. The last three pitches of
> [measure 1] do reference three of the four pitch classes involved; to that degree there is
> a certain amount of closure. The F#, G, and C# that one hears there finally summon the
> C at the flute entrance in m. 6 (436–37).

In Lewin's writing, two complexes of metaphors have clustered around inversional symmetry. The first imagines the state of inversional balance as a harmonious ideal, one that can be challenged, disrupted, or obscured, and possibly reestablished. The second has to do with the desire imputed to musical tones to find their inversional partners. And the two metaphors are closely related: the desire of individual tones to form inversional partnerships is a manifestation of a more global musical interest in establishing, or reestablishing, inversional balance.

To grasp the full impact of these metaphors, it is important not to overlook their physicality, their origins in bodily experience. Most people have bodies that are symmetrical and depend on that symmetry for the maintenance of physical balance. If the symmetry is disrupted, the resulting loss of balance may be experienced as challenging, disruptive, frightening, and potentially catastrophic. The persistence of imbalance may be experienced as a disabling condition, an impairment that prevents normal, smooth navigation through the world. In that situation, a person's physical experience of asymmetry and imbalance in his/her own body may be like Schoenberg's view of musical imbalance—a problem to be solved, a restoration and recuperation to be desired, a disability to be overcome.

To that extent, Lewin's transformational theory exemplifies the normalizing thrust of traditional music theory. But unlike the form theorists and Schenker, Lewin is not at heart a conformationist or a normalizer. He is not concerned about what most pieces do and is not at all fearful (as Schenker is) about what might happen if works deviate from the norm. For him, imbalance is neither stigmatized as a problem nor celebrated as an inspired deformation. Rather, the process of moving in and out of a state of balance is worthy of attention for its own sake. The musical processes (transformations) lead where they will in response to local musical conditions, unconstrained by any master narrative. The body is still at issue, but its variations are purged of both stigma and special artistic value.

In a field where so much has traditionally depended on sorting the normal from the abnormal, Lewin thus stands out for his resistance to what Scully (2008, 4) calls "the therapeutic imperative." For Lewin, the goal of music theory and analysis is not to situate deviations as deficits or excesses with respect to some norm; rather, the goal is to individuate pieces, to tailor a theory-of-the-piece that makes the piece most itself. In this sense, Lewin's transformational theory is transformational not only in its attitude toward musical structures but also in its attitude toward the disabled musical body.

CHAPTER 7

Performing Music and Performing Disability

MODES OF PERFORMANCE

Musical performers have extraordinary bodies, capable of supranormal skill, dexterity, strength, and memory. Compared to the general population, or even the smaller population of music lovers and amateur music makers, top musical performers are prodigious figures. When unusual musical abilities become apparent in a young child, we call him or her a "prodigy," suggesting both the rarity of the gift as well as its affinity with monstrosity—a shocking deviation from normative embodiment.[1]

If musical performers have extraordinary, prodigious, even monstrous bodies, then musical performances have an aspect of a freak show: audiences pay to see and hear unusual figures whose appearance and ability deviate far from the norm. In exchange for the price of a ticket, audience members can stare (and listen intently), indulging in the simultaneously disquieting and reassuring contemplation of a human embodiment so like and yet unlike their own.[2]

---

1. According to the *Oxford English Dictionary*, a prodigy can be "an unusual or extraordinary thing or occurrence; an anomaly; something abnormal or unnatural; *spec.* a monster, a freak" as well as "a person with exceptional qualities or abilities *esp.* a precociously talented child." Garland-Thomson (2009, 163–64) elaborates the relationship between the prodigious and the monstrous:

> Monsters are unusually formed beings whose bodies are simultaneously ordinary and extraordinary.... The long history of monster and freak shows offers the most florid example of how and why people look at dissonant shapes and scales.... Monstrous bodies were a particular type of prodigy—similar to comets and earthquakes—which drew great attention and inspired awe.

2. The freak show has attracted considerable attention from scholars of disability (see Bogdan 1988; Garland-Thomson 1996; and Adams 2001). Freak shows involve a process of "enfreakment"—the constitution of an unusual body as a deviant Other:

For musical performers with visible (or audible) disabilities, the affinity between a performance and a freak show may become even more pronounced.[3] Musical performers are subject to the same disabilities that everyone else is, although these may have particular effects on musical performance, such as pianist Paul Wittgenstein's loss of an arm to a war wound (Howe 2010b) or jazz guitarist Django Reinhardt's loss of two fingers on his left hand in a fire. These would be disabilities in almost any context, but they take on particular significance in the face of the technical demands of a musical instrument. Furthermore, there are disabilities that are music-specific—bodily differences that become disabilities only in a musical context. I am thinking, for example, of focal distonia (uncontrollable muscle contractions, often in the hand, that affected pianists Leon Fleischer, Gary Graffman, and many others) or vocal disfluency (damage to the vocal chords that may affect singing, but not normal speech).[4] The more comprehensive music-related disability of *amusia*—known more familiarly as "tone deafness"—is worthy of serious study not only from experimental psychologists but also from disability scholars, but it is unlikely to play a role in high-level musical performance (see further discussion in chapter 8).

For performers with visible disabilities, audiences come not only to hear the music but also to stare at the disabled body: the blind or mad or one-armed pianist, the guitarist with three fingers, the singer with vocal damage, the violinist with polio, the deaf percussionist. In such situations, the disabled performer has a dual task: to perform music and to perform disability.[5] The idea that disability is not so

---

At the same time that enfreakment elaborately foregrounds specific bodily eccentricities, it also collapses all those differences into a "freakery," a single amorphous category of corporeal otherness. By constituting the freak as an icon of generalized embodied deviance, the exhibitions also simultaneously reinscribed gender, race, sexual aberrance, ethnicity, and disability as inextricable yet particular exclusionary systems legitimated by bodily variation—all represented by the single multivalent figure of the freak. Thus, what we assume to be a freak of nature was instead a freak of culture. The freak show made more than freaks: it fashioned as well the self-governed, iterable subject of democracy—the American cultural self. Parading at once as entertainment and education, the institutionalized social process of enfreakment united and validated the disparate throng positioned as viewers. A freak show's cultural work is to make the physical particularity of the freak into a hypervisible text against which the viewer's indistinguishable body fades into a seemingly neutral, tractable, and invulnerable instrument of the autonomous will, suitable to the uniform abstract citizenry democracy institutes (Garland-Thomson 1996, 10).

3. The relationship between the body and musical performance—the conceptualization of musical performance as in some sense embodied—is a growing area of study in the field of musicology (see, for example, LeGuin 2006). The bodies in question, however, are generally idealized and always fully capable. The disabled body has not been theorized in relation to musical performance.

4. On dystonia see Sacks (2007) and Woo (2010). On vocal disfluency, see Stras (2006).

5. For an important discussion of these issues in music from an insider perspective, that is, from a musical performer with a visible disability, see Honisch (2009), who argues that the concert hall "forces audience and performer alike to reflect on how ability and disability are contiguous phenomena, continuously playing against each other."

much a static quality that inheres in a body but more a performance has become familiar in Disability Studies, as it did previously in gender studies and queer theory.[6] Like gender and sexuality, disability is not something you are, it's something you do.[7]

Within a social or cultural model, disability is understood as constructed rather than given—it emerges from the activities of human beings in relation to each other and to the culture and built environment they inhabit, not from the medical pathology of an individual body. If disability is constructed, then it is constructed by people who are doing something, and their actions constitute a performance. To perform disability is to construct it, and vice versa.

For people with disabilities, the performance of disability is a constant feature of daily life; through their actions, they show the normal world what a disability is and what it means to live with one. As Davidson (2008, 18–19) argues,

> From nineteenth-century freak shows and carnival acts, through the photographic displays of eugenics textbooks to Jerry Lewis telethons, disability has been synonymous with the theatrical display of "different" bodies. At the most immediate level, disability

6. The idea of gender as performative rather than inherent is most closely associated with Judith Butler. As White (2003, 137) summarizes:

> Butler does not accept what seems obvious on the face of it: there are two opposite sexes; sex is a natural cause of desire; gender is the inevitable expression of a natural, underlying, biological sex. Rather, she turns her attention to how sex, gender, and desire are culturally and discursively constructed in this way, how they are made to take their place in the heterosexual matrix and then are naturalized.... Butler argues that any genuinely nonhegemonic resistance to the regime of compulsory heterosexuality must seek to deprive it of its essential (and essentialized) protagonists: "man" and "woman." Her project is to render the very idea of gender incredible. Dismissing the notion that gender somehow expresses biological sex, she reconceptualizes gender as the performative effect of reiterative acts. Gender is thus constituted by the very expressions that are said to be its results. The performance of gender is not a volitional act but is compelled by the regulatory practices of gender coherence, and those who fail to perform their gender properly are regularly punished. Compulsory and repetitive performances of gender create the idea of gender, and without them there would be no gender at all.

See Butler (1993, 1999).

7. As Sandahl and Auslander (2005, 10, 215) contend,

> To think of disability not as a physical condition but as a way of interacting with a world that is frequently inhospitable is to think of disability in performative terms—as something one *does* rather than something one *is*.... Part of sociology's legacy to performance studies is the idea that we do not just live our "real life" identities, we *perform* them.... Goffman argues that who we are socially is bound up with who we are perceived to be by those around us (our audience) and that we behave as actors in order to control the impressions we make on others. This understanding of everyday behavior emphasizes that identity does not simply reside in individuals but is the product of social interactions among individuals. This perspective is congruent with the view of disability as something that is not an intrinsic characteristic of certain bodies but a construct produced through the interaction of those bodies with socially based norms that frame the way those bodies are generally perceived.

is constructed through complex rituals of staring and avoidance that occur when people confront a person with an empty sleeve, a prosthetic limb, a scarred face, a stutter. These social pragmatics are double-edged: the able-bodied viewer averts the gaze or looks clandestinely, the disabled subject "performs" invisibility—acts as though invisible or else compensates in some way to make the viewer feel comfortable. Disability memoirs are filled with descriptions of what we might call crip double consciousness in which the individual in a wheelchair must simultaneously "act normal" while negotiating an inaccessible and sometimes hostile environment. The late actor and playwright John Belluso, who used a wheelchair, describes the theatricalization of disability as a continuous public performance: "When I get on a bus, all the heads turn and look, and for that moment, it's like I'm on a stage. Disabled people understand the world in a different way. You understand what it's like to be stared at, to be looked at, and in a sense you're always performing your disability."[8]

In many cases, the performance of disability is designed to make the nondisabled feel comfortable, at ease, unthreatened, as Garland-Thomson (1997, 13) suggests:

> Disabled people must use charm, intimidation, ardor, deference, humor, or entertainment to relieve nondisabled people of their discomfort. Those of us with disabilities are supplicants and minstrels, striving to create valued representations of ourselves in our relations with the nondisabled majority.... If such efforts at reparation are successful, disabled people neutralize the initial stigma of disability so that relationships can be sustained and deepened. Only then can other aspects of personhood emerge and expand the initial focus so that the relationship becomes more comfortable, more broadly based, and less affected by the disability.

For musical performers with disabilities it becomes imperative to find a way of presenting their disability in a nonthreatening way—to neutralize it for their audience. Failure to do so may result in what Garland-Thomson (1997, 11) describes as "engulfment," that is, a process wherein a person is reduced to their disability, "stripped of normalizing contexts and engulfed by a single stigmatic trait".[9]

If neutralization does not seem possible, a musical performer may try to pass as nondisabled. Or, to put it another way, a musician with a disability may try to perform ablebodiedness. This will be a good deal easier, of course, if the disability is invisible. The opposite of passing is the affirmative claiming of disability, what Tobin Siebers calls "disability as masquerade": "The masquerade counteracts passing,

---

8. Likewise, Sandahl and Auslander (2005, 1–2): "Disability in daily life is already performance.... In daily life, disabled people can be considered performers, and passersby, the audience."

9. Likewise, see Kuppers (2001, 49–50) on the power of cultural narratives to preempt whatever a disabled artist might be attempting to communicate: "When disabled people perform, they are often not primarily seen as performers, but as disabled people. The disabled body is *naturally* about disability."

claiming disability rather than concealing it. Exaggerating or performing difference, when that difference is a stigma, marks one as a target, but it also exposes and resists the prejudices of society" (Siebers 2008, 118). In this sense, performers with disabilities may claim disability as an affirmative part of their identity, a defining part of the self that they perform (along with the music they perform) for their audience.

In some cases, the masquerade may even become a marketable "shtick," part of what audiences find attractive. In most spheres of life, disability entails severe, negative economic consequences. In the world of performance, and under certain circumstances, the masquerade of disability may confer economic benefits. In a situation like this, audiences come to hear a performance not despite the performer's disability but precisely because of it; they seek the pleasures of staring.

As Garland-Thomson (2005, 31) observes, staring is "the dominant mode of looking at disability in this culture," and "the normative stare constructs the disabled." Disabled artists, including musicians, perform their art and their disability simultaneously. For people with disabilities, then, performance on a stage is a concentrated dose of the transactions of daily life—the disabled performer invites and challenges the normate stare.[10]

The musical performer is a "staree," in the formulation of Garland-Thomson (2009), someone with an extraordinary body who simultaneously invites and shapes the staring encounter:

> Because lived staring encounters are spontaneous and dynamic, they can be pliable under the guidance of an experienced staree. Indeed, accomplished starees often develop a repertoire of strategies they use to choreograph staring encounters.... Stareable people have a good deal of work to do to assert their own dignity or avoid an uncomfortable scene. People with unusual looks come to understand this and develop relational strategies to ameliorate the damage staring can inflict. Rather than passively wilting under intrusive and discomforting stares, a staree can take charge of a staring situation, using charm, friendliness, humor, formidability, or perspicacity to reduce interpersonal tension and enact a positive self-representation (8, 84).

Performers with disabilities "stage a dramatic encounter by inviting the staring that objectifies their bodies and then orchestrating that performance so as to create the

10. The term "normate" is a neologism of Rosemarie Garland-Thomson's, designed to suggest that normality, like disability, is a social construction:

> This neologism names the veiled subject position of cultural self, the figure outlined by the array of deviant others whose marked bodies shore up the normate's boundaries. The term *normate* usefully designates the social figure through which people can represent themselves as definitive human beings. Normate, then, is the constructed identity of those who, by way of the bodily configurations and cultural capital they assume, can step into a position of authority and wield the power it grants them (Garland-Thomson 1997, 8).

image they intend to project. It is the task that all disabled people face writ large" (Garland-Thomson 2005, 33). Just as people with disabilities learn through daily experience to manage the social interactions that are initiated by staring, the disabled performer stages the staring encounter.[11]

As noted earlier, the available roles for the performance of disability are somewhat limited and fall into certain predicable categories, which Sandahl and Auslander call "cultural scripts" (Sandahl and Auslander 2005). Norden (1996) describes some of these scripts as they play out in film, and observes that disabled people in film are usually depicted as Obsessive Avengers, Sweet Innocents, Comic Misadventurers, Noble Warriors, Saintly Sages, High-Tech Gurus, Tragic Victims, or other stereotypical roles. A more general typology of disabled roles in literature is offered by Leonard Kriegel (1987, 33):

> It is the diseased and afflicted [who] impose their presence on the "normals." In showing themselves, they call attention primarily to their wounds. At its most gripping and perhaps memorable, this is done in the wild, sustained manner such as Shakespeare's Richard and Melville's Ahab. But the Demonic Cripple as embodied in Richard and Ahab is only one corner of the box. Along with him, we have the cripple as victim, or the Charity Cripple ... the cripple whose wound is merely a part of his overall sense of selfhood—the Realistic Cripple ... and the cripple who triumphs not over but against misfortune by outlasting the effects of his wound until those effects have been incorporated into his way of dealing with the world—the Survivor Cripple.

To Norden's film roles and Kriegel's Demonic, Charity, Realistic, and Survivor Cripples, I would add two additional categories. First, the Natural Man or Woman is a person whose disability seems to strip him or her of any civilized veneer, lowering him or her to the level of a brute beast. A literary prototype might be Shakespeare's Caliban, whose outward disfigurement is an emblem of his inner depravity. As we shall see, musical performers with disabilities are often understood in this light, and the beautiful music they produce is seen as profoundly incongruent with their misshapen, deformed bodies. Second, the Mad Genius is a person whose cognitive impairment or psychological disturbance is bound up with a super-

---

11. Likewise, see Ferris (2005, 56–57):

> Awareness of fictionality is an essential component of aesthetic distance, a concept that provides some explanation for how we know the difference between what happens on the stage, for example, and real life. This is, of course, quite different from an awareness of the fictionality of disability. But disabled performers, through the management of aesthetic distance, may be able to expose the fiction of disability, transforming the closed look of the stare into a more open look that is both receptive and creative.... Distance— both physical and emotional—is a factor in any relationship between people. The concept of aesthetic distance can illuminate the negotiations and implications involved in the management of physical space and interpersonal distance and show ways disabled people can manage their own performances to redefine the stare and present themselves as real people while not minimizing their experiences of oppression.

human vision. As with some of the composers discussed in chapter 1, their madness is taken as an emblem of their genius. To some extent, musical performers choose among these roles and present themselves in one of these interpretations of disability even as they present their interpretations of the musical works they perform.

To these typologies of disability performance, Garland-Thomson (2001) adds a useful typology of disability reception, what she calls "a taxonomy of four primary visual rhetorics of disability: the wondrous, the sentimental, the exotic, and the realistic" (339). Each of these rhetorics suggest a way in which audiences might respond to the sight of a visibly impaired performer: "the wondrous mode directs the viewer to look up in awe of difference; the sentimental mode instructs the spectator to look down with benevolence; the exotic mode coaches the observer to look across a wide expanse toward an alien object; and the realistic mode suggests that the onlooker align with the object of scrutiny" (346). These are modes of audience response and therefore are only partly under the control of the performer. Nonetheless, performers may choose to push the audience in one or more of these directions.

People with disabilities, provided they have decided not to try to pass and the disability is visible or can be made visible, have some degree of latitude (within culturally defined limits) as to the way they perform their disability. In what follows, I will describe the ways in which a selected group of performers with disabilities perform their music and their disabilities, and the ways in which these two types of performances intertwine and inform each other. For a performer with a disability, public musical performance is usually understood as inherently a triumph over adversity, and such performances are normally assimilated to familiar narratives of overcoming. My interest, however, is not in showing what these performers can do in spite of their disability, but rather what their disability enables them to do.

A full-scale study of musical performers with disabilities would have a vast terrain to cover. Internationally, many countries have long traditions of musicians with disabilities, especially blindness. And within popular traditions in the West, the number of performers with disabilities, again especially blindness, is extremely large.[12] A quick, superficial survey would include exemplary figures such as José Feliciano, Ray Charles, Stevie Wonder (Hughes 2003), Joni Mitchell,[13] Connie Boswell,[14] Mel

12. See Rowden (2009) and a special issue of *Popular Music* (28/3 [2009]) devoted to popular music and disability.
13. Joni Mitchell had polio as a child, and its lasting effects limited the range of movement in her left hand. Her disability shaped her writing and her playing in this very direct way, circumscribing the kinds of chords she could play on the guitar and therefore the kinds of chords she wrote. See Sonenberg (2003).
14. Connie Boswell (1907–76) was an important and influential jazz singer and a frequent musical partner with Bing Crosby. Paralyzed from the waist down by childhood polio, her disability affected both the reception of her singing (her preferred medium, radio, made concealment possible) and the singing itself. See Stras (2009).

Tillis,[15] Greg Saunier,[16] Rick Alten,[17] The Blind Boys of Alabama, Django Reinhardt,[18] and many others. The Western classical tradition of musical performance—the focus of this chapter—is equally rich in performers with disabilities of every kind, especially blindness. In what follows, I will consider closely a small handful of musical performers in the Western classical tradition whose lives and music-making (including its reception by audiences and critics) have been definitively marked by disability.

THOMAS WIGGINS ("BLIND TOM")

Thomas Wiggins (or Thomas Bethune), widely known as "Blind Tom," was one of the most famous musicians in the nineteenth-century United States. Born a slave in Georgia in 1849, Wiggins was apparently autistic as well as blind, and probably intellectually disabled as well. He emerged as a skilled improviser and composer and, to judge from his performance repertoire, a highly accomplished pianist. His concerts were spectacles, designed to showcase his remarkable talents. Over the course of an evening, he would play works from the standard piano repertoire, including some that posed significant technical challenges, some parlor songs, and some of his own compositions, all from a repertoire of several thousand works played from memory upon request. In addition, he would perform prodigious feats of musical memory and coordination, including playing back any work upon hearing it for the first time, simultaneously playing two different songs (one with each hand) while singing a third, and identifying all of the notes in complex harmonies.[19] Throughout his

15. Mel Tillis is an American country music singer with a significant stutter.
16. Greg Saunier, the drummer for the Deerhoof, has Tourette's Syndrome.
17. Rick Alten, the drummer for Def Leppard, has only one arm.
18. Django Reinhardt, the early jazz guitarist, was badly burned in a fire in 1928 and lost the use of two fingers in his left hand. According to James (2001), this "led him to devise a unique fingering method to overcome his handicap." See also Dregni (2004).
19. Here is one contemporary account, from the *Fayetteville Observer* (May 19, 1862), written by correspondent Long Grabs:

> The blind negro Tom has been performing here to a crowded house. He is certainly a wonder.... He resembles any ordinary negro boy 13 years old and is perfectly blind and an idiot in everything but music, imitation, and perhaps memory. He has never been instructed in music or educated in any way. He learned to play the piano from hearing others, learns airs and tunes from hearing them sung, and can play any piece on first trial as well as the most accomplished performer.... One of his most remarkable feats was the performance of three pieces of music at once. He played Fisher's Hornpipe with one hand and Yankee Doodle with the other and sang Dixie all at once. He also played a piece with his back to the piano and his hands inverted. He performs many pieces of his own conception—one, his "Battle of Manassas," may be called picturesque and sublime, a true conception of unaided, blind musical genius.... This poor blind boy is cursed with but little of human nature; he seems to be an unconscious agent acting as he is acted on, and his mind a vacant receptacle where Nature stores her jewels to recall them at her pleasure.

concerts, Wiggins displayed unusual verbal and physical behaviors, talking about himself in the third person, pacing and spinning around, flicking his fingers, singing, humming, grunting, and making unusual facial gestures.[20] His concerts were extremely popular public spectacles, part musical entertainment, part freak show (O'Connell 2009; Southall 1979, 1983, 1999; Jensen-Moulton 2006; Rowden 2009).

It would be hard to imagine a more fascinating nexus of race, disability, and musical performance. For the white observers of his day, Wiggins was taken as an epitome of what was most degraded, bestial, and inhuman about the "Negro race"—in this way his disabilities and his race are intertwined as aspects of his defective "otherness." From a more current perspective, Wiggins might be better understood as typifying an autistic approach to music ("autistic hearing" will be discussed in detail in chapter 8).[21] One aspect of autistic music-making is the preference for hearing musical events in relative isolation from each other and from any subsuming context—a radically piecemeal, nonrelational way of approaching music. This would seem to have been a unifying feature of many of Wiggins's most remarkable abilities, including his absolute pitch, his ability to play unrelated musical works simultaneously, and his ability to memorize musical nonsense (for nonautistic listeners, memorative ability falls off sharply in the absence of normative networks of musical relationships). Autism is not directly visible; rather, it must be made evident through certain kinds of behavior, both verbal and physical. By performing music in this manner, and accompanying the musical performance with characteristically autistic behaviors—talking to himself, nonverbal vocalization, spinning in circles, stereotypical hand and arm gestures—Wiggins performs his disability.

Wiggins's extensive concert tours of the United States and Europe (including a concert at the White House for President Buchanan) were widely covered in the press. Observers were struck most by the incongruity of the spectacle: beautiful, highly cultivated music emerging from a monstrous, uncivilized body. Indeed, that incongruity was the essence of Wiggins's distinctive appeal, and as he presented himself to the public marketplace (and as he was presented by his handlers), it was in his (and their) financial interest to emphasize that incongruity. Southall (1999)

---

20. As Jensen-Moulton (2006) shows, many of Wiggins's verbal and physical behaviors are typical of autism. Rowden (2009, 28), however, contends that Wiggins's mannerisms are "blindisms":

> An especially significant aspect of the illusion of privacy that the congenitally blind are actively taught to recognize and control is the public display of those mannerisms that in blindness research have come, albeit problematically, to be called "blindisms." Although Tom's mental impairment is undeniable, his seemingly uncontrolled physical gestures, rather than being evidence of his "idiocy," may simply have been blindisms generated by his congenital sightlessness.

21. Three recent accounts that place Wiggins on the autism spectrum are Jensen-Moulton (2006), Davis and Baron (2006), and O'Connell (2009).

argues that the extent of Wiggins's intellectual disability may have been exaggerated by his managers for commercial purposes and by the contemporary press for the sensationalism of an "idiot" with such astonishing musical gifts. By "enfreaking" him, Wiggins's managers situated him as an embodiment of widely circulated cultural stereotypes of both disability and race (Rowden 2009). This is a slightly different sense of performing disability, as Wiggins may have deliberately enhanced his disability to increase his market appeal.

Wiggins performed his disability in conformity with well-established cultural scripts, and the role he adopted has aspects of the Saintly Sage, the Sweet Innocent, the Comic Misadventurer, the Demonic Cripple, and above all, the Natural Man—brutish and uncivilized. One aspect of the mythology around Wiggins, cultivated by his managers, was his complete lack of formal musical training. Wiggins was portrayed as innocent of the cultivated tradition; his musical performances were therefore spontaneous, instinctive, and miraculous. This is entirely false. In fact, Wiggins throughout his life had instruction and coaching from well-trained musicians and mastered his craft as all musicians do, through extensive guided practice (O'Connell 2009).

Another related myth was that Wiggins played perfectly and that his musical memory was beyond comprehension and explanation. In fact, according to the best-informed listeners and most knowledgeable insiders, he was an excellent pianist, but with some technical limitations, and his memory, although remarkably good, fell within the range of other equally gifted musicians. Wiggins was neither a Sweet Innocent nor a Natural Man, but rather an immensely gifted musician whose musical performances and performances of disability were confined to narrow cultural scripts. Following those scripts, Wiggins's performances often involved low comedy. As a Comic Misadventurer, he played his disability (and his race) for laughs, according to the conventions of the minstrel show.[22]

Audience members sometimes understood Wiggins as a kind of Saintly Sage, one whose disability is an external marker for divine inspiration:

> We see this awkward and stupid Negro led to the piano stool; he takes the seat, but the first touch on the keys shows us his soul is made for music. He sweeps his hands over the keys with the air of a master and then we behold the inspiration manifesting itself in his countenance and movement…. An ecstatic influence flows from the keys into his fingers…. A light kindles the blank face and, as we gaze, wondering, the fashion of his countenance seems to change. It is absolutely beautiful. This divine ravishment increases every moment and, when he is thoroughly suffused with the inspiration of the melody, the muscles in his face twitch and his upper teeth are placed firmly upon his lower lip (review from the *Charleston Courier*, quoted in O'Connell [2009, 81]).

22. The stereotypical conjunction of disability and race, in which each is used to intensify the stigma attached to the other, and both are played for crude laughs, may account for Wiggins's lack of appeal for black audiences, even after emancipation (Rowden 2009). Wiggins's performances were shaped by his white managers for the entertainment of a white audience.

Listeners like this one were responding in wondrous or sentimental mode. Exotic mode, however, was a much more common response: observers cast him as a deeply alien monstrosity. Mark Twain, Wiggins's most famous admirer, was almost overwhelmed by the incongruity of a saintly, innocent angel trapped within the body of a monstrous brute:

> All the schooling of a life-time could not teach a man to do this wonderful thing, I suppose—but this, blind, uninstructed idiot of nineteen does it without any trouble. Some archangel, cast out of upper Heaven like another Satan, inhabits this coarse casket; and he comforts himself and makes his prison beautiful with thoughts and dreams and memories of another time and another existence that fire this dull clod with impulses and inspirations it no more comprehends than does the stupid worm the stirring of the spirit within her of the gorgeous captive whose wings she fetters and whose flights she stays. It is not Blind Tom that does these wonderful things and plays this wonderful music—it is the other party ("Letter from Mark Twain," *The Alta California*, August 1, 1869).

Similar themes preoccupy lesser-known critics: a spark of the divine buried within a demon; a monstrous incongruity of childlike innocence and gross physicality; a stark clash of civilized beauty and frightening, untamed nature; and, in some cases, a sense of comedy in Wiggins's "antics."[23]

> Some curious metaphysical questions grow out of these remarkable demonstrations. What is this boy? A negro—belonging to an unintellectual race; himself an idiot. But what is intellect and what is idiocy? Can he be an idiot with whom those achievements are most ordinary which in others are pronounced the grandest evidences of masterly genius? And what is it to be "developed"? Where is the narrow dividing line that separates the philosopher from the fool? Here is a monstrosity—a gorgon with angel's wings; a sunflower with the blush of a mignonette and the fragrance of a mountain rose. There is no law by which to measure and determine such exhibitions as this (*Albany* (N.Y.) *Argus*, January 1866).
>
> For some time past the wonder-seekers of London have been amused by a series of performances, vocal and on the pianoforte, by a negro boy called Blind Tom. The boy, *who is not only blind, but completely and unmistakably idiotic*, executes *difficult* music with a facility that under the circumstances is remarkable, and goes through several feats which rather indicate mnemonic and imitative powers than a genius for music, properly so called. Thus, while he plays *one air with his right hand* he accompanies it by *another air in another key with his left*, and *sings a third air in a third key at the same time*, thus giving a specimen of a school of harmony which is peculiar to himself.... Even while he is

---

23. The critical responses to "Blind Tom" quoted below may be found in "Opinions of the English and American Press," *The Black Perspective in Music* 4/2 (1976): 180–83.

displaying his peculiar gifts, the appearance of utter idiocy remains; his face goes into curious contortions when his notes become more than commonly expressive, and by clapping his own hands he responds to the applause of the audience. (*Times* [London], August 18, 1866).

We were quite prepared from the metropolitan press to find in Blind Tom some extraordinary qualities, fortified as their statements were by the testimony of M. Moscheles, who tested the alleged powers of this nigger youth at Southsea, and publicly expressed his opinion that Tom was "marvelously gifted by nature." After hearing him last night at the Theatre Royal we can most consciously endorse this opinion; but to give in writing anything like an accurate description of him is utterly impossible. The fingers fly over the keyboard, and he seems like one possessed. Did not Shakespeare conceive this being when he describes Caliban being touched with the magical sounds heard in Prospero's Island?...Behind that strange visage, and underneath that imperfectly organized brain, what is going on? We dare not speculate. He is evidently a freak of nature, but he must be heard and seen to be in any degree comprehended (*Manchester Guardian*, September 26, 1866).

The critics were overwhelmed by Wiggins's disabilities, and by the perceived contrast between his disabilities and his musical gifts.[24] He had the appearance of a freak, a monster, a gorgon, and one normally expected such obvious bodily difference to be a mark of inward deformity as well—Wiggins looked like an Obsessive Avenger. But within his hideous form lurked the soul of an angel, a mountain rose. In other words, he was a Sweet Innocent, whose musical gifts are too pure, too refined, too good to be explained in any rational way. His bodily difference was thus a mark of his spiritual superiority. But whether his body signified his satanic or angelic nature, it always signified, and it always engulfed Wiggins the musician, Wiggins the pianist, and Wiggins the composer.

In "Blind Tom" we find an unusually gifted musician—performer, improviser, composer—whose visible disabilities (blindness, autism, and, to most of his contemporary white critics, African ancestry) entirely engulfed critical response. For normatively embodied observers (sighted, neurotypical, white), his music-making, down to its smallest detail, was understood in light of his disabilities. The music and the disabilities were intertwined, and the audience wanted to see extravagant performances of both.

GLENN GOULD

Glenn Gould (1932–1982) is generally acknowledged as one of the greatest pianists of the twentieth century. He performed and recorded widely, both as a soloist

24. Additional critical responses to "Blind Tom," thematically similar to these, may be found in Riis 1976.

and with major orchestras, and left a legacy of audio and video recordings that are still very much in demand. As a pianist, he is best known for the astonishing clarity of his playing—each line and each note sharply etched—and for the shocking originality of his musical interpretations. As a performer, he is at least equally well known for his many eccentricities: he sat very low at the piano, and accompanied his playing with constant singing and humming, as well as unusual hand gestures; he was a germ-phobic hypochondriac, who always wore an overcoat, even in the summer; his personal grooming was below normal standards. He disliked the give and take, the socially interactive nature, of live performance and, at a relatively early stage in his career, he permanently left the concert hall for the privacy and seclusion of the recording studio. For many critics, their annoyance at Gould's unusual behaviors engulfed their response to his music; they found it impossible to talk about the music without reference to the behavior. Even among Gould's supporters, and he has by now achieved something like cult status among classical music lovers, a big part of the allure was his obvious deviance from normal standards of behavior for pianists. Like the audience who went to hear "Blind Tom," Gould's listeners are drawn both to the music and to the strange personality.

It has recently been argued, convincingly in my view, that Gould belongs on the autism spectrum, and that his autism provides a common source both for his personal eccentricities and his distinctive musical interpretations.[25] His profound social disengagement—the hallmark of autism—isolated him not only from the live concert audience but also from the community of past and present pianists. His autism may thus have contributed to the astonishing originality of his interpretations.

Specific aspects of Gould's playing may also be related to his autism, including his preference for the extreme isolation of individual tones through persistent *staccato* articulation. One of the distinctive features of Gould's playing is separation and detachment: he separates the lines within a polyphonic texture, and within each line he separates the notes from each other.[26] The detachment of lines from other lines, and notes from other notes, is a striking musical affirmation of an autistic

25. Maloney (2006, 134) persuasively places Gould on the autism spectrum through careful study of the extensive written and video archive:

> Autism is the solution to the perplexing riddle of [Glenn] Gould's existence and is therefore arguably the fundamental story of his life. It leads us to a coherent understanding of both the man and the musician. Not only does it gather all his strange behavioral and lifestyle eccentricities into a unified *gestalt*, it also furnishes intriguing insights into important aspects of his music-making.

Autism remains a controversial issue in Gould studies. Ostwald (1997) is a psychobiography that raises but does not pursue the issue of autism. Bazzana (2004) discounts autism, preferring instead a mixed account based on anxiety, depression, hypochondria, and "a variety of obsessional, schizoid, and narcissistic traits" (370).

26. According to Bazzana (1997, 215–16), "As a general rule, Gould preferred articulation that can best be described as non-legato or détaché.... His desire for clarity, so basic to his musical personality, extended to his rendering of phrases and even individual notes.... Détaché was the norm for Gould regardless of tempo."

preference for "local coherence."[27] In this sense, Gould's autism provides a way of understanding his life and his art in an integrated way. Instead of seeing his famous "eccentricities" as distracting, inessential personal mannerisms, we can see them as part of an autistic worldview. By behaving as he does, and by playing as he does, Gould performs his autism. Gould performs his disability largely as a Saintly Sage, one whose musical ability has something otherworldly about it. The response to him has accordingly typified Garland-Thomson's "wondrous mode," as audiences have looked up at Gould "in awe of difference."

THOMAS QUASTHOFF

Internationally acclaimed bass-baritone Thomas Quasthoff was born in 1959 as, in his words, "one of twelve thousand thalidomide children" (Quasthoff 2008, 35). In a cultural environment hostile to people with visible physical disabilities, Quasthoff faced severe difficulties in obtaining the sort of education and musical training to which his intelligence and musical talent would entitle him. He was initially forbidden to attend a mainstream school: "Father appealed to the education authority, approaching even the minister of education. The answer was always the same: Cripples are not welcome. Cripples belong in a special school" (54). Eventually he did attend a regular school but, after his musical talent became evident, he was refused admission to the Music Academy in Hanover:

> I complete an application but don't hear anything for weeks. When the deadline for matriculation has almost passed, Father reaches for the phone. He will not be deterred, not by the president's secretary nor by Professor Jacobi. But the head of the academy is an arrogant man who refuses to discuss the matter. He won't even let me audition. "Dear man, the German academic regulations require command of at least one instrument— the piano." "But I already told you he is a thalidomide child with maimed arms." "And if I understood you correctly, your son is—for whatever reason—not capable of doing so, which is why he will not be accepted here. And I tell you right now he will not be accepted elsewhere either. Good-bye" (Quasthoff 2008, 88).

Despite these early setbacks, Quasthoff did manage to receive an appropriate musical training followed by performance opportunities in increasingly prestigious settings. He is now widely recognized as one of the preeminent classical music

27. In one currently prevalent theory of autism, it is seen as a disorder characterized by "weak central coherence"—an atypically weak tendency to bind local details into global percepts. In this view, the deficits in social relatedness, as well as other intellectual deficits associated with autism, are manifestations of an underlying inability to create larger meanings or social patterns from discrete elements (see Frith and Happé 1999; Frith 2003; and Happé 2005). Autism in relation to a predilection for local coherence will be further discussed in chapter 8.

vocalists of our time. The trajectory of his life and career can thus be easily assimilated to traditional disability narratives of overcoming: the triumph of the human spirit over adversity.

That familiar trope of disability heroically overcome also provides the subtext, or the explicit text, for critical reception of Quasthoff's singing. A typical example comes in an article from *Time Magazine*, titled "Triumph of the Spirit: German Singer Thomas Quasthoff is Thrilling Audiences with his Voice—and his Courage":

> Like thousands of other German women in the late 1950s and early '60s, Quasthoff's mother took thalidomide as a sedative during her pregnancy. As a result, Quasthoff, 37, stands about four feet tall, and as is common for thalidomide victims, he has severely underdeveloped arms and hands which emerge almost directly from his shoulders. All of this is, of course, immediately obvious when he walks onto a stage and perches on a platform that puts him level with the other performers. But almost from the instant Thomas Quasthoff begins to sing, all audience awareness of his disability simply melts away. "With him on the one hand you have the quality of the voice, and on the other hand, his great musicality, with which he makes the work his own," says Helmuth Rilling, the director of Stuttgart's International Bach Academy and a conductor who has engaged Quasthoff for many appearances over the past few years. "I find it unjust to say it's astonishing how this man with his handicap can sing so beautifully. One must say [the handicap] has nothing to do with it" (Gleick 1997).

Not surprisingly, this is not a critical approach that Quasthoff likes. Indeed he resents finding his artistry and his disability endlessly juxtaposed:

> The writers bring out the big guns when they want to connect my singing with my unorthodox appearance. "He did not let himself be disabled" is one of the more subtle lines, "Disability is no obstacle" or "Disabled takes all hurdles," and "Disabled with superb voice." The unsurpassed classics remain: "The handicapped dwarf Quasthoff limped across the stage and illuminated Paulus" and the one I already mentioned, "He sings as if God wanted to correct a shop accident" (Quasthoff 2008, 143).

Like many artists with disabilities (and like artists belonging to any oppressed minority group), Quasthoff expresses the desire to have his art appreciated on its own terms: he wants to be appreciated as a singer, not as a disabled singer. In a recent interview, Quasthoff expressed the desire for a shift of critical attention from his disability to his art, to avoid being engulfed by a stigmatic trait.

> If performing live on national television represents a career milestone for Mr. Quasthoff, is it also a breakthrough for people with deformities? Asked if he sees himself as a role model, Mr. Quasthoff said, "If it's true, it's a nice side effect." But the danger of

focusing on this, he added, is that he could start to play a role as a representative for the disabled. The only role he wants to play, he said, is that of "serious artist" (Tommasini 2004).

In his public statements, Quasthoff does his best to downplay the role of disability in shaping his life and career. In the process, he sometimes seems to disavow his kinship with other disabled people and to assert that his art permits him to transcend this stigmatized category:

> For me, my disability is a fact and not a problem. I'm not living the life of a disabled person. For sure, I have to handle some things differently from other people. But it's not so different from the life of someone who is not disabled. In any case, who is really not disabled? I am in the lucky position that everyone can see it. But if you are never happy, if you are only concerned about money or success, this is in my opinion also a kind of disability (Quoted in Moss 2000).

When Quasthoff says, "I'm not living the life of a disabled person," he is imagining the extremely difficult and narrow circumstances under which most people with disabilities, in Germany perhaps more than in the United States or the UK, are forced to live (Poore 2009).

Quasthoff is fully aware of the extent to which he is exceptional among people with disabilities. His talent and his luck have permitted him to escape what would have been a more likely fate in a punishingly ablist culture. With regard to an invitation to a television talk show in 1992, he writes:

> Of course, it was not really music they wanted to hear about but thalidomide and a human being who refused to let even the most severe disability spoil his good mood. My excitement was limited. I was familiar with this story of the happily chirping pill victim, and while it is true that I am no weeping willow, I do not like being presented as a model handicapped person. I am not a role model or a life counselor, and I am not here to assuage the guilt of a society that equips certain office buildings with special entrances but otherwise punishes its physically incapacitated with constant disrespect. What good are my experiences for someone with a thalidomide disability if he cannot sing, or paint like Picasso but with his mouth? No good at all. Less spectacularly disabled people still have a hard time finding employment.... Most of the disabled population is left to vegetate on welfare, or packed away in homes and exploited as cheap labor. Thank God, I was able to flee this ghetto after my ninth birthday—thanks to the loving care of my parents, my musical talent, the tolerance of a select few, and a lot of luck. I therefore find it hypocritical to join an organization for the disabled and make thalidomide the central fact of my life. Unlike most of those who share my fate, I have had the opportunity simply to accept my physical deficits as fact, much as others see their bunions, even if it was a long and painful process. The reader who has followed me patiently up to this point knows that I have not led a typical disabled life. I got the same smacks on the head as my brother, had the same normal friends, the same

problems and formative experiences.... When press, radio, and television come at me with the old handicap stories, I now find it exhausting and growl my standard sentence: "I am one of eighty million disabled Germans—I just happen to be more visible" (Quasthoff 2008, 204–205).

These remarks reveal an interesting ambivalence. Because of his exceptionality (due both to his celebrity and his largely mainstream upbringing and education), he would find it "hypocritical" to act as an advocate for disability rights. At the same time, he has a strong sense of identification with the larger disability community, and a profound anger at the injustices it experiences.

These comments represent a rare outburst of anger from Quasthoff. For the most part, his public personality is easygoing, sunny, and relentlessly cheerful. I take this as Quasthoff's chosen way of managing social interactions with the non-disabled. He seeks to disarm their fears by concealing his anger. He is no Obsessive Avenger or Demonic Cripple, full of resentment against an unjust world, in search of revenge against his oppressors. Rather, he's just a regular guy—cheerful, friendly, unthreatening. In this way, he seeks to "neutralize the initial stigma of disability" (Garland-Thomson 1997, 13).

In common with other performers with disabilities, Quasthoff's critical reception often focuses on an apparent incongruity between his physical appearance and his art. In the case of "Blind Tom," the notable incongruity was between his demonic, deformed appearance and the angelic purity of his music. In Quasthoff's case the comparable incongruity is between the diminutive size of his body and enormous size of his voice. Quasthoff himself is fully aware of the centrality of this trope in his critical reception. Here is his description of one of his early public concerts:

> The audience did in fact whisper and look rather dumbfounded. But that's no surprise—they've never seen anything like me on a concert stage before. A Lilliputian tot without arms, jerking around in front of the podium because his legs are squeezed onto splints. But as soon as my baritone rolled through Carl Loewe's majestic ballad "Prinz Eugen" there was silence in the auditorium. It soon became amazement, and by the end it was sheer enthusiasm. No doubt they felt as if they were watching a bit of magic. No one expects so many rabbits to fit in a top hat. No one expects such a mighty voice to issue from my diminutive frame (Quasthoff 2008, 91).

Similar responses pervade even the most recent criticism.

Many reviews depict Quasthoff as a kind of Saintly Sage, one whose obvious bodily differences and presumed suffering have conferred upon him a superior, visionary knowledge. His disability is understood as an outward marker of his deep inner wisdom.

> Quasthoff at 42 is on the hero's path of adventure through rites of passage, in a process defined by the late Joseph Campbell, heading towards—perhaps already arriving

at—transfiguration. He is no longer "just a singer," not even if called, justifiably, a great, unique one. He has transformed into a kind of cultural icon, the classical-music equivalent of Elvis, the Beatles and the Rolling Stones put together. He makes a difference in people's lives, with his artistry, palpable joy in music and life, personal example of overcoming unimaginable hardship and challenges with grace, courage and a kind of seductive elegance. And, most importantly for an artist, Quasthoff brings these elements into his work, instead of allowing them to become fodder for tabloids (Gereben 2002).

Like Landini's blindness and Beethoven's deafness, Quasthoff's "birth defects" are emblems of an enhanced interiority. His presumed suffering sets him not only apart from normal people, but above them, engaging Garland-Thomson's "wondrous mode."

Quasthoff himself is much more circumspect in identifying ways in which his disability has affected, possibly benefited, his musical interpretations.

I am in the good position of not being able to make gestures with my hands so my voice is the only form of expression that I have. This forces a huge concentration on the part of the audience. If you remain still and have only the face and the voice, the audience has to concentrate, much more so than for those who use gestures. So maybe it is also an opportunity (Quoted in Moss 2000).

One area in which Quasthoff's disability might have a direct effect on his music is that of operatic roles. Quasthoff was long reluctant to sing opera because of its physical demands, and opera houses were extremely slow to offer him roles because of his appearance. That has changed a bit in recent years, but the roles offered most often have been those of disabled operatic characters.

I have received many offers from large houses already and have always declined. I haven't felt mature enough, and it seems an unnecessary display of my disability....I must ask myself whether I really have enough acting talent and physical presence for it, for despite Simon [Rattle]'s encouragement the fear of exposing myself to ridicule still gnaws at me....I liked the part of Amfortas right away because of its singable character, very unlike Verdi's crippled Rigoletto, for example, which I had been offered frequently but which I did not want to sing (Quasthoff 2008, 127–28, 129, 135).

This raises interesting questions. On one hand, in a world of operatic casting that is willing to suspend disbelief when it comes to race, age, and various other physical characteristics, one would like to see Quasthoff offered the full range of operatic roles to which his voice is suited. On the other hand, his portrayal of Amfortas—the suffering, wounded king in Wagner's *Parsifal*—takes on a special resonance in Quasthoff's performance, and it is probably an improvement of the pervasive practice, in film and theater as in opera, of having able-bodied performers appear as disabled characters.

ITZHAK PERLMAN

Itzhak Perlman occupies an almost unique position in our culture, a classical musician (acknowledged as one of the greatest violinists of our time) and a popular celebrity. He also has a visible disability, namely a mobility impairment resulting from polio, which he contracted at the age of four. Since then, Perlman has worn leg braces. He has generally gotten around using crutches and plays the violin in a seated position. In more recent years (Perlman is now 63), his mobility has become further impaired by post-polio syndrome and he has come to rely more on a scooter or wheelchair, although usually not in a public performance.[28]

Like Quasthoff, Perlman's accounts of his childhood emphasize its relative normality, and his sense of gratitude that he was not shunted aside into the sorts of ghettos often reserved for people with disabilities:

> My parents were very supportive in a normal way. It was never: "Oh, we have a child who has polio!" They were naturally instinctive parents who did things not just by the book, but by feel.... With my childhood friends, the abnormal thing about me was not that I walked with crutches—they got used to that. The abnormal thing about me was that I had to practice three hours a day. The other kids thought that was crazy (Larkin 1986).
>
> I lived in a house, I had friends, I played hide-and-seek, I went to school like everyone else, and I had a lot of fun. I liked school very much. And, until I turned thirteen, that was my childhood. You can make a normal situation out of an abnormal situation very, very easily. It has to do with how you are treated and what you are able to do. In my case, this [i.e., polio] never interfered with anything (Nupen 2007).

Perlman was a childhood prodigy. After a series of early successes in his native Israel and elsewhere, Perlman became an overnight celebrity when he appeared on the Ed Sullivan Show at the age of thirteen, and has been a universally acclaimed public figure since then. Early critical accounts situated his playing in relation to his disability and traced a familiar narrative of overcoming—the brilliance of his playing comes in spite of his disability and represents a triumph over disability:

> [Perlman is a] 13-year-old Israeli violin prodigy who has overcome the crippling handicap of polio to become one of the world's most promising musical artists (*Los Angeles Times* 1958; author unknown).
>
> The soloist was the 22-year-old Itzhak Perlman, whose mastery of the violin and development of artistry extraordinary for one so young have been achieved despite a crippling attack of polio when he was 4½ years old (Hughes 1968, 26).

---

28. Rothstein (1993) claims that Perlman uses a motorized wheelchair in his private life.

> Crippled by polio before he was five, this young man has practiced and performed his way to the top of his field (Hughes 1969, 34).

> A childhood bout of polio left him unable to walk without leg braces and crutches. But it did not stop him from going on to become one of the most highly prized artists of his generation (Kriegsman 1971, B1).

Perlman has reacted strongly against critical reception in this vein. For a long time he considered it demeaning to be identified in terms of his disability and resented any inference that his successes came either in spite of or, even worse, because of his disability:

> When I first played Carnegie Hall at 17, one reviewer said he wasn't sure if the standing ovation I got was because I played well—or because I was disabled....Many people questioned whether or not I could have a career....At the time, I didn't understand that at all. I just thought maybe I should practice harder (Quoted in Larkin 1986, N3).

> It used to bother me. Like, you know, the headline on the review "Polio Victim Stars in Violin Concert"—that kind of thing. There was one incredible one, I remember: "Mr. Perlman hobbled out on the stage, and his aluminum crutches glistened through the orchestra." Wow! (Quoted in Henahan 1970, D15).

For a long time, Perlman did not welcome discussions of his disability, which he considered peripheral to his core concerns as a musician. He has often used humor as a way of deflecting questions about disability and of defusing any concerns about the sort of vengeful anger that the able-bodied so often impute to the disabled. Rather than an Obsessive Avenger or Demonic Cripple, he wishes to appear genial, affable, generous, and open-hearted:

> Asked if the affliction had caused him to devise any special approach to his instrument, he replied with a smile, "No, not at all. The only thing I can say it has done for me is that I won't have to apologize in my old age for being flat-footed" (Kriegsman 1971, B1).

More recently, as he has become increasingly active as an advocate for the disabled and especially for architectural accessibility, Perlman has changed his attitude. Now, instead of attempting to distance himself from his disability, he actively claims it as a core part of his identity:

> At the beginning of my career, the critics always mentioned my disability—the headlines would say something like, "Crippled Violinist Plays Concerto"—and that made me mad. Now they never mention it and I *want* them to. I think it is important to identify myself not only as a violinist but as one who has a disability (McLellan 1981, D1).

Perlman now speaks frequently about issues of accessibility in travel, lodging and concert halls, using his celebrity to advance the cause of social justice:

Architects can improve one negative aspect that people with disabilities must face: eliminating architectural barriers. But unfortunately architects are not educated in barrier-free design (Quoted in Larkin 1986, N3).

A lot of people think access means the ability to get into a building, no matter where or how you can get into it, whether you get into it through a back alley, or through an elevator that usually carries garbage or food. But shouldn't it mean you can get into the building through the front door with everybody else? That for me is true access (Quoted in Rothstein 1993, R1).

I have begun refusing to play in some halls because of access problems—for the audience or for me (Quoted in McLellan 1981, D1).

I travel in a narrow space. My world is composed of concert halls, hotels and airports. They can be inaccessible in all sorts of ways....Whether I'm walking on crutches or in a chair, the architectural barriers are the next big problem [after attitudinal]. The theatre in Haifa won a big architectural award. But there are steps everywhere. So finally I made my entrance one night and said, "I'm playing this concert under duress. I'm never playing here again unless you put an elevator in." Now there's an elevator. It's in the back, but goddamn it, it's an elevator—the Perlman elevator.... In Amsterdam there's this wonderful hall which is world famous, the most wonderful acoustics there are. I don't play there anymore. They have 25 steps in view of the audience to reach the stage. I always felt I was performing twice when I played there. First I was performing by everyone following me up the steps, "There he goes—the first step! There he goes—the second step! Here he comes...will he make the fourth step?! He slipped, oh no, there he is, the sixth step! Oh, he made it!!" Then they will clap with relief when I finally appear on stage. Then I had to play (Quoted in Lewis 1981, 11).

Although Perlman has claimed disability in a notably forthright and politically effective way, it will be interesting to see the extent to which he acknowledges his increasing use of a scooter and a wheelchair in his public performances. At present, Perlman still comes on and off stage using crutches despite using a scooter or a motorized wheelchair in more private settings. Visual images of Perlman, including video images, almost universally show him seated—he is rarely depicted with crutches or seated in a scooter or wheelchair. If he were to use his scooter or wheelchair on the concert stage, that might be a potent statement of affiliation and support for the larger post-polio community. It would also be a further move toward encouraging audience response in a realistic rather than a sentimental mode.

EVELYN GLENNIE

Evelyn Glennie is a young Scottish percussionist who has had remarkable success and recognition. She is probably the first percussionist in the classical tradition to achieve international stardom. She has performed with major orchestras, commissioned and premiered dozens of new works, and received extensive media coverage and rapturous reviews. She is a remarkable musician of extraordinary charisma and originality.

Glennie lost much of her hearing when she was twelve years old, and her deafness has affected her music-making and its reception in profound ways. In her own account of her development, Glennie (very much like Quasthoff and Perlman) emphasizes the normality of her upbringing:

> Growing up with my parents and two brothers in a farm outside Aberdeen, Scotland, I was never treated as a special case. Part of the reason was that my parents didn't know how to treat me any differently, but also because life just went on normally as it did after I lost my hearing. Why should it suddenly change when, at age twelve, I lost my hearing? What was so important about my upbringing was how normal it all was.... Everybody just acted normal, which was the best thing that could have happened (Reisler 2002, 43).[29]

At every stage, however, Glennie's deafness has shaped the way she makes sense of music and produces music, causing her to attend to the tactile and visual aspects of sound: she feels and sees the music.[30]

> Deafness is poorly understood in general. For instance, there is a common misconception that deaf people live in a world of silence. To understand the nature of deafness, first one has to understand the nature of hearing. Hearing is basically a specialized form of touch. Sound is simply vibrating air, which the ear picks up and converts to electrical signals, which are then interpreted by the brain. The sense of hearing is not the only sense that can do this, touch can do this too. If you are standing by the road and a large truck goes by, do you hear or feel the vibration? The answer is both. With very low frequency vibration the ear starts becoming inefficient and the rest of the body's sense of touch starts to take over. For some reason we tend to make a distinction between hearing a sound and feeling a vibration, [but] in reality they are the same thing.... Deafness does not mean that you can't hear, only that there is something wrong with the ears. Even someone who is totally deaf can still hear/feel sounds.... So far we have the hearing of sounds and the feeling of vibrations. There is one other element to the equation, sight. We can also see items move and vibrate. If I see a drum head or cymbal vibrate or even see the leaves of a tree moving in the wind then subconsciously my brain creates a corresponding sound (Glennie 2010a).

29. Likewise, see Glennie (1990).
30. A tactile way of hearing is reflected in the titles of a documentary film about Glennie, "Touch the Sound" (Riedelsheimer 2004) and her autobiography, *Good Vibrations* (Glennie 1990).

By attending in her performances to the sights and feelings of the sounds she hears and produces—she performs barefoot and with extraordinary visual intensity—she makes her deafness visible to the audience, simultaneously performing her music and her deafness.

Glennie's deafness has inflected and threatened to engulf critical response to her work. Virtually every review refers to it and virtually every interviewer asks about it. Some of the critical response has positioned her as a Saintly Sage. In a distant echo of the Wagnerian understanding of Beethoven's deafness, Glennie's deafness is seen as isolating her from the dirty world of music commerce, positioning her above the daily fray. More commonly, she is described as a Natural Woman, whose disability frees her from the normal conventions of civilized society. In many cases she is seen as a bit of both—her deafness is both a source of higher vision and a mark of her position outside normal society: "Glennie doesn't simply play the music, she becomes the music, transmitting it to the audience like some sort of feral nature priestess" (Carol Simmons, *Dayton Daily News*, November 2001).

Glennie has made it clear repeatedly that she does not want to talk about her deafness any more, that she considers it an irrelevance and a distraction.

> To summarize, my hearing is something that bothers other people far more than it bothers me. There are a couple of inconveniences but in general it doesn't affect my life much. For me, my deafness is no more important than the fact I am a 5'2" female with brown eyes. Sure, I sometimes have to find solutions to problems related to my hearing and music but so do all musicians.... Please enjoy the music and forget the rest (Glennie 2010a).

Glennie argues that whatever she has achieved has come not in spite of deafness (the familiar narrative of overcoming) or because of it (an activist stance of claiming disability). Rather, her deafness has had no significant impact:

> I have truly never believed that the problems I experienced with my ears could in any significant way affect my abilities as a musician. Neither did I believe that just because no one else had ever succeeded in maintaining a career as a solo classical percussionist that I would not be able to. I have not succeeded in spite of my deafness or because of it. Deafness is simply an irrelevant part of the equation. For instance some of the things I do when playing would be a lot easier if I had longer arms and bigger hands. So I could consider this as a physical handicap. Compared to the general consensus concept of arms and hands though, mine aren't particularly out of the ordinary so rather than dwell on my physical inadequacies I simply find a workaround. Certainly my hearing is out of the ordinary as others might see it, but not for me it isn't. I'm used to my hearing in the same way that I'm used to the size of my hands (Glennie 2010b).

Glennie argues that her deafness is now irrelevant because it has been overcome: her career represents a triumph over an obstacle. With reference to her autobiography (Glennie 1990), she says, "I hope that *Good Vibrations* will show that it is possible to succeed with one's ambitions, despite apparently almost insurmountable obstacles" (11). Her story, as she tells it, is "the story of a little girl growing up on a farm in Scotland, determined against all the odds to make a life in music" (19).

But it cannot be denied that Glennie's deafness has added to her appeal and to her celebrity. Part of the public's fascination with her is directly attributable to her deafness. People want to come and stare and be astonished. As with "Blind Tom" and Thomas Quasthoff, the public enjoys the sense of incongruity between an "extraordinary body" and the kind of music that would seem to be incompatible with it. Without any effort on Glennie's part, and in fact in spite of her resistance, her deafness has been an important part of her box office appeal.

Beyond questions of economics, Glennie's deafness is integral to the way she understands and makes music. Even while proclaiming its irrelevance, Glennie acknowledges that her deafness not only shapes her music, but does so in advantageous ways:

> So is hearing loss ever an advantage? In my situation, it's an advantage because it allows me to put my stamp on the interpretation of the music. I don't rely on recordings to know how a piece should go. Most people do, because it's a quick way to learn a piece. But I have to learn the full score and basically read it. So, everything I do is entirely mine, whether you like it or not, which I think in the long run, is a tremendous advantage because it gives me confidence in what I want to say. There are no rules at all (Reisler 2002, 49).
>
> I never hoped that they would discover some miraculous cure for my hearing.... It didn't disappoint me to learn that no surgery or hearing aid currently available was going to restore me to good hearing. I had learnt to cope with my silent world, and felt that my own ways of listening to music gave me a sensitivity that I far preferred to the "normal" way of hearing that I had experienced as a tiny child. Because I had to concentrate with every fibre of my body and brain, I experienced music with a profundity that I felt was God-given and precious. I didn't want to lose that special gift (Glennie 1990, 125–26).

At moments like this, Glennie comes very close to claiming deafness as a positive identity, at once artistic, cultural, and social.

For the most part, Glennie has held the Deaf community at a distance. She has been a committed oralist, and has expressed concern that Deaf institutions and Sign Language are intrinsically and undesirably isolating. Recently, however, Glennie's views seem to have moderated. In 2008, she announced that, at the age of 42, she had begun to learn Sign Language: "I've only now thought about what sign language really means, what it is, and what I feel it can bring to my particular situation. Like any language, it takes time and consistency and that's our challenge at the moment because we don't have consistent time" (Macaskill 2008). It will be interesting to see whether or not this signals a change in Glennie's attitude toward her deafness and toward the Deaf community. If it does, perhaps Glennie will learn new ways of performing her deafness even as she continues to evolve as a performer of music.

CHAPTER 8
Prodigious Hearing, Normal Hearing, and Disablist Hearing

WAYS OF HEARING MUSIC

This chapter turns from composers and performers to listeners with disabilities, and consider the possibility that differences among bodies—differences in morphology and functioning that may be classified as disabilities—might shape the way people make sense of music. Traditional music theories of the kind surveyed in chapter 6 assume an extravagantly gifted listener, an expert trained to hear the sorts of complex musical relationships modeled by the theory. Listening to music in the manner of Schoenberg, Schenker, Hepokoski and Darcy, and Lewin requires *prodigious hearing*. The relatively new field of music cognition, in contrast, both describes and enforces *normal hearing*. That is, music cognition enshrines a notion of how people who are understood as normal—physically, psychologically, and cognitively—make sense of music. Normal hearing also lies at the core of music pedagogy: in our universities and schools of music, we teach students to hear normally.

In opposition to the normalizing impetus of music cognition, with its unexamined reliance on the normal listener, and to the sorts of normal hearing we customarily teach our students, I propose what I will call *disablist hearing*: the ways that people whose bodily, psychological, or cognitive abilities are different from the prevailing norm might make sense of music.[1] If "situated knowledge adheres in

---

1. A word about terminology. The terms "disability" and "disabled" are inherently problematic, with their inescapable connotations of deficit and defect. There is no neutral larger category within which "disabled" could be a marked term, that is, no term analogous to gender as a category that embraces both male and female. As a result, "disability" has to do double duty as both the overarching category and one of the specific terms, where it stands in opposition to "normatively abled." Likewise, there is no good term for the prejudice and negative stereotypes that have always surrounded people with disabilities (analogous to racism or sexism). The most common term is "ableism," although some sources (mostly in the UK) use the term "disablism." In using the term "disablist" here, I intend an analogy to the term

embodiment," in Tobin Siebers's (2008, 23) pithy phrase, then we might expect people with disabilities to hear music in ways that differ from the norm. Disablist hearing, habitually and unconsciously excluded from music-theoretical discourse and from prevailing models of musical perception and cognition, offers an alternative to prodigious hearing and normal hearing.

MUSIC THEORY AND PRODIGIOUS HEARING

Music theories typically construct models of musical structure, explicitly or implicitly contrasting normal and abnormal structures. Since the early nineteenth century, music theory has taken as its project the establishment of statistically normal harmonic progressions, contrapuntal combinations, and formal patterns as a standard against which to measure deviance. In this sense, traditional music theory is essentially a normalizing enterprise, and thus bound up with the medical model of disability (as discussed in chapter 6).

Although music theory has traditionally focused on structures within the music itself, it nonetheless also conveys at least an implicit sense of what a musical listener is or should be. Each theory imagines—effectively calls into being—a suitable listener. For the most part, the implicit listeners in traditional music theory are prodigious figures, with extensive training and vast knowledge of the musical literature. These listeners use their extraordinary abilities to classify musical forms, separating the norms from the deformations (in the manner of Hepokoski and Darcy), to create networks of musical motives over various spans of time and in various presentations, demonstrating how deviant and problematic elements are subsumed within a normative frame (in the manner of Schoenberg), to create structural hierarchies in which dissonant or chromatic elements are heard in relation to consonant, diatonic norms at all levels of structure (in the manner of Schenker), and to apprehend inversional symmetry operating in complex transformational networks (in the manner of Lewin). Listening of this kind could be called "theoretical listening," that is, listening for the sorts of relationships that have been of interest to music theorists.[2]

To be able to hear in this way requires rare musical abilities and intensive musical training. These prodigious listeners are far from normal, indeed, they are almost as rare as composers and performers of the first rank. As Schenker (1997, 8) observes,

---

"feminist," and I describe a mode of hearing associated with disabled people, but not necessarily confined to them.

2. Compare Adorno's (1988, 4–5) "expert listener" who "tends to miss nothing and at the same time, at each moment, accounts to himself for what he has heard." According to Adorno, such listeners are so few in number as to be "probably scarcely worth noting." The distinction I am making between prodigious and normal hearing resonates with a related distinction made by DeBellis (2002, 130) between "structural hearing" and "intuitive hearing," also referred to as "ordinary cognition" and "the ordinary listener's pretheoretical, intuitive hearing."

I am keenly aware that my theory, extracted as it is from the very products of artistic genius, *is and must remain itself art,* and so can never become "science." While in no sense a scheme for breeding up geniuses, it does address itself primarily to practicing musicians, and only the most gifted of those, at that. Capable though it is also of liberating music theory, history, aesthetics and philosophy from centuries-old errors, it really only addresses such representatives of those branches of knowledge as possess the highly-developed musical ear demanded by the art of genius. Since this theory revolves primarily around the concepts of composing-out and diminution, and is concerned on the creative side with artistic invention in accordance with Nature, and on the recreative or listening side with empathetic artistic response, it is a totally closed book to all those incapable of discerning such purely compositional phenomena.

The implied listeners in traditional music theory inhabit prodigiously capable bodies (they have great ears, as musicians say). In most traditional music theories, listeners are encouraged to normalize what they hear, that is, to distinguish the abnormal elements (e.g., problematic notes, dissonant harmonies, formal deviations) from the normal ones, and to understand the former in relation to the latter. However, prodigious hearing may also encompass marvelous, fantastic, or arcane musical relationships—prodigious listeners may hear things in music that normal listeners do not.

MUSIC COGNITION AND NORMAL HEARING

The relatively new field of music cognition shifts attention from musical works to the listener and asks how listeners make sense of music. Instead of describing musical structures, music cognition seeks to describe the cognitive basis for our musical perceptions and intuitions, grounding them in the "unchanging cognitive foundations of the musical mind" (Lerdahl 2001, vii).[3] Music cognition studies listeners using the methods of experimental psychology, including a reliance on

---

3. Lerdahl (2001, vii, 4) writes:

> I have endeavored to develop a framework for understanding music that incorporates both the relatively unchanging cognitive foundations of the musical mind and the historical continuities that underlie changes in musical style.... [Lerdahl and Jackendoff 1983] treats music theory as the branch of theoretical psychology concerned with modeling the musical mind.... The strategy is to isolate the spontaneous musical cognitive capacity as an idealized object of study.... To assert that a rule is universal is to claim that it represents a natural propensity of the musical mind.

One finds similar general statements throughout the literature. See, for example, Temperley (2007, 5): "The underlying aim is to uncover the mental processes and representations involved in musical behaviors—listening, performing, and composing." Serafine (1988, 233) understands music as a form of cognition and contends that "the artform is not considered a clearly specified external object, but rather an internal, subjective entity springing from mental operations."

statistical analysis. Even more than traditional music theories, then, music cognition is a normalizing enterprise: it creates and depends upon normal listeners hearing normally.

Who are these listeners? The normal listener, as far as experimental psychology is concerned, is usually an undergraduate student at a research university in the United States; these individuals make up the vast majority of the experimental subjects. Obviously, these listeners are chosen for study for a practical reason: they are readily available to researchers. I would suggest that there is also another reason: they are selected because of their normal embodiment—they are physically, psychologically, cognitively, and intellectually normal.[4] As a result, researchers assume that their subjects may be taken as representative of human beings in general.[5]

Having first selected subjects because of their normative embodiment, the studies proceed as if differences in embodiment were irrelevant (the scientific method requires that we strip away as much personal and musical context as possible). As a result, the listening subjects, chosen for their particular bodies, are strangely disembodied. The unexamined insistence on homogeneous subjects, whose individuality and bodily variation has been systematically repressed, necessitates the exclusion of large classes of people whose embodiment differs from the norm.

What sorts of musical abilities do these listeners have? The listeners who are included in psychological studies have either no formal musical training or just enough to qualify them as "experienced" listeners. Usually, an experienced listener is someone with some degree of formal musical training (either instrumental lessons or college level courses), the ability to read music notation, and some knowledge of the relevant musical repertoire (usually the works of the classical tonal canon). As the famous opening sentence of Lerdahl and Jackendoff (1983) states: "We take the goal of a theory of music to be a *formal description of the musical intuitions of a listener who is experienced in a musical idiom*" (1). The authors go on to observe,

---

4. As Krumhansl (1990, 5–6, 9) explains:

> Cognitive psychology is a subarea of experimental psychology concerned with describing human mental activity.... The cognitive psychologist is generally less concerned with the occasional exception or special case than with the more general rules governing human cognition. Furthermore, the focus is less on describing the experience of specially trained or exceptional individuals than with cognitive capacities exhibited more generally.... Because cognitive psychology is directed at describing mental capacities exhibited quite generally, the majority of studies do not employ participants with extraordinary talents or severe deficits.

5. Indeed, these studies require that the subjects be fungible, somewhat in the manner of industrial workers—that is, they are replaceable parts in the machine. Individual differences are not of particular interest and, as in the workplace, they are typically unaddressed and unaccommodated (O'Brien 2005).

The "experienced listener" is meant as an idealization. Rarely do two people hear a given piece in precisely the same way or with the same degree of richness. Nonetheless, there is normally considerable agreement on what are the most natural ways to hear a piece. A theory of a musical idiom should be concerned above all with those musical judgments for which there is substantial interpersonal agreement (3).

Thus, studies of music cognition exclude prodigious listeners, those whose extraordinary musical gifts place them near one edge of the bell-shaped curve of musical abilities. We understand that such people hear in highly individual, even eccentric, ways. Their hearing is not representative of normal musical cognition.[6]

At the other edge of the bell-shaped curve of musical abilities, studies of music cognition exclude people who are incapable of cognizing the simplest kinds of musical relationships. Traditionally, we tend to refer to such people as "tone-deaf." In a culture that routinely medicalizes variation in human abilities, such people are now classified as having the disorder of "amusia."[7] These studies also exclude people whose physical or intellectual differences impinge on their cognition of music, including, for example, listeners who are autistic, hearing impaired, or visually impaired. In short, they exclude anyone whose hearing is not normal, that is, not characteristic of the large majority of modestly skilled college students.

Under what circumstances do these normal listeners listen? In the psychological experiments that form the basis for music cognition, listeners are typically alone in a cubicle listening to a sound source through headphones. They hear alone, without seeing the performers of the music they hear, and without the possibility of responding kinesthetically to what they hear (i.e., singing, playing, or dancing). What they hear tends to be isolated snippets of sound, divorced from any larger musical context. This decontextualization is intrinsic to the scientific method with its attempt to control the variables under study. It does, however, mean that normal hearing takes place in a strangely unnaturalistic environment, a problem of which

6. As Butler (1992, 6) observes: "Psychologists tend to be interested in testing perceptual theories that generalize to a large segment of the world population, while musicians tend to be interested in learning more about the expert musical behaviors practiced by competent, well-trained musicians—a fairly small segment of the general population."

7. For an overview of the literature on amusia, defined as "acquired clinical disorders of music perception, performance, reading, or writing that are due to brain damage and not attributable simply to the disruption of basic perceptual, motoric, or cognitive functions," see Marin and Perry (1999, 655). See also Ayotte, Peretz, and Hyde (2002). Sacks (2007) identifies many different kinds of amusia, including receptive amusia, interpretive amusia, performance amusia, rhythm deafness, tone deafness, true tone deafness, gross tone deafness, total amusia, acquired amusia, congenital amusia, complete congenital amusia, pure pitch amusia, gross dystimbria, dysharmonia, and cochlear amusia. According to Sacks, "One speaks of an amusia when the perception of some or all of these qualities [tone, pitch, timbre, loudness, tempo, rhythm, and contour] is impaired" (144).

music psychologists are well aware.[8] Not only is normal hearing strangely disembodied, it is also ahistorical and asocial. Most of the music under study was composed during a period when music-making was a participatory, social activity. Even setting aside the technological anachronism for 18th- and 19th-century music of its dependence on recorded sound, normal hearing is radically different from historically informed or authentic listening practices.[9]

What sorts of musical relationships are these normal listeners presumed to be listening for? Studies of music perception have been almost exclusively concerned with relations among pitches. The sorts of subtle timbral and articulative relationships that typically preoccupy performers play little or no role. Beyond the most basic aspects of pitch, studies of music perception have been interested in the ways listeners make sense of musical pitch structures like melody, harmony, rhythm and meter, voice leading, and form, topics that have traditionally been of interest to music theorists. For higher-level constructs of this kind, there seems to be a consensus among music cognitionists that listeners hear hierarchically, with similar processes operating over different spans of time, the smaller nested inside the larger.[10] Serafine (1988, 233) considers hierarchic levels as one of a "set of cognitive processes thought to form a core of understanding common to composing, performing, and listening."[11] Other researchers generally concur:

> Listeners seem to be able to form patterned groupings of tones on several different bases. Pitch proximity is one common and powerful basis of perceptual grouping: listeners will sort tones into separate groups according to their registral proximity and/or their melodic coherence, and will even ignore strong cues for location and timbre when they conflict with the perceptual imaging of reasonable pitch patterns. Melodic groupings can be nested within one another, sometimes resulting in complex hierarchical arrangements (Butler 1992, 125).

8. Butler (1992, 6) identifies this as "the most troublesome methodological dilemma in music perception research" and observes, "The more control we gain over the auditory stimulus, over the listening environment, and over the response task, the more music we must take out of both stimulus and response."

9. This observation is original with Blake Howe (personal communication).

10. The consensus is not complete, however, and Sloboda (2005, 139) offers a caution about the psychology reality of hierarchies:

> Because hierarchies are so appealing they bring with them a danger. People tend to impose hierarchical explanations to an extent that may be inappropriate. In particular, what works well at a local level may not necessarily translate to higher levels, and vice versa. There is a satisfying elegance to complete hierarchic descriptions of entire pieces of music (such as those supplied by Schenker [1979] and Lerdahl and Jackendoff [1983]), but many observers, including psychologists, have pointed out that the ability to describe something in hierarchic terms does not necessarily mean that listeners represent what they hear according to such descriptions.

11. See also Bharucha and Krumhansl (1983).

We have provided evidence that memory for pitch and for low-level pitch relationships is based on a number of highly specialized systems, and that at higher levels pitch information is retained in the form of hierarchies (Deutsch 1999, 403).

The core aspect of tonal cognition is to perceive which tones anchor which tones.... Organizing the pitch events of a piece into a single coherent structure, in such a way that the pitch events are heard in a hierarchy of relative importance, is the most fundamental aspect of tonal cognition for Western music (Bigand and Poulin-Charronnat 2009, 59–60).

The most vigorous statements on the subject come from Lerdahl and Jackendoff (1983, 280): "Musical intuitions are organized along the four hierarchical dimensions treated here: grouping, metrical structure, time-span reduction, and prolongational reduction. Each of these (with specified exceptions such as overlaps) is a strictly hierarchical structure that includes every pitch-event in the piece." In the world of music cognition, Lerdahl and Jackendoff's has long been the most prevalent theoretical model of traditional, classical tonal music and its cognition.[12] For most researchers, then, the cognition of tonal structures is hierarchical in nature.

We are now in a position to summarize the principal features of normal hearing. It is associated with cognitively and physically normal American college students with modest musical training and ability. It is undertaken in isolation from other people and without the possibility either of seeing the performed source of the sound or of responding to the sound kinesthetically. Finally, normal hearing is focused on pitches, which it organizes hierarchically. In each of these respects, normal hearing—despite its pretensions to universality—presents at best a partial and exclusive picture of human music cognition.

Normal hearing is described and enforced by current studies in music cognition, but it is not created there. Rather, it is a mode of hearing that is taught in our music studios, classrooms, and schools. Only recently have we begun to offer meaningful accommodations to students with disabilities, especially cognitive or developmental disabilities, and as a result our students are mostly nondisabled. When we play a recording for our students, or ask them to notate a melody we play for them, or engage in much of the typical business of a music classroom, we ask them to respond individually, without assistance or collaboration, without seeing the

12. As Cook (1994, 71) observes, "A cursory survey of current writing in music psychology might suggest that [Lerdahl and Jackendoff 1983] is the dominant model in tonal music theory, almost to the exclusion of any other." Lerdahl and Jackendoff's intellectual project is nicely summarized in Klumpenhouwer (2005, 489):

> Their goal was to define the theory of music held (unconsciously) by the perception system of experienced listeners to tonal music. The working out of these ideas had a number of different dimensions, two of which deserve special mention: first, a belief in the hierarchical nature of cognition; and second, a commitment to the idea that the relevant cognition is innate.

performed source of the sound, and without permitting audible or kinesthetic response. We focus attention on pitch relationships, especially the possibility of hearing hierarchically, creating groups out of individual pitches, and then larger groups out of smaller ones. In all of these ways, we teach normal hearing.

And it is usually not an easy process. It requires extensive, repetitive drill, hard and concentrated work, constant pushing and prodding. Normal listeners are not given, they are created, and it the job of music teachers to create them. There is nothing natural about normal hearing; rather, it is a cultural artifact, the end result of a long and sometimes arduous process of acculturation. When the process of acculturation is sufficiently advanced, a student may be certified as an "experienced listener" and thus a suitable subject for a study of cognition. Such a study may then claim to be describing the "unchanging cognitive foundations of the musical mind," but that is an illusion. Music cognition purports to discover natural and universal ways of understanding music, but more likely it merely reflects back to us the results of our teaching.

Compared to prodigious hearing, normal hearing is less elitist, more democratic and widespread, more inclusive. Lots of people have the ability to be normal listeners. And it is in the nature of music cognition studies, as it is in the nature of music pedagogy, to aim for the large middle, by lopping off hearings (and listeners) who are either strange and marvelous (prodigious) or judged defective in some way. That is inherent in these enterprises, and it is hard to see how they could do things differently. The problem is not so much that music cognition and music pedagogy focus on normal hearing, but rather that they pretend to naturalness and universality. In fact normal hearing and normal listeners, like all kinds of hearing and all kinds of listeners, are made by culture, not given by nature.

DISABLIST HEARING

Until the present moment, the music-making of people with disabilities (including people with physical, cognitive, or intellectual impairments or psychological disorders) has been largely confined to two intellectual ghettos. The first ghetto is that of "abnormal psychology." Within the psychology literature, one finds case studies of the music-making or music cognition of people with disabilities, and I will sample some of this literature below. For the most part, however, the subjects are discussed exclusively in terms of their disability, that is, their musicianship is understood as fully circumscribed by their disability; it does not represent the generic human norm. The distinctive cognitive abilities, including musical abilities, of people with autism, for example, have been widely and intensively studied, but always in isolation from the normal mainstream.

Within musical scholarship, disabled listeners are relegated to a second intellectual ghetto: music therapy. According to the goal statement of the American Music Therapy Association, music therapy "is an established healthcare profession that uses music to address physical, emotional, cognitive, and social needs of children and adults with disabilities or illnesses." In other words, music therapy is a normalizing enterprise, bound up with the medicalization and attempted remediation of disability. Of course there is a long history stretching back to classical antiquity of accounts of the power of music to cure or disable.[13] What's new in the field of music therapy is the full impact of the medical model of disability: its practitioners are medical professionals who offer therapy to patients and write up their findings in the form of case studies. They seek to cure, remediate, or normalize their patients, and music is their therapeutic tool.[14]

Under the music therapeutic regime, the listener is a medical patient, a recipient of care. The listener is defined in advance as defective—physically, cognitively, or socially—and the goal of the therapy is to provide treatment.[15] To the extent that music therapy encourages and enables music-making, it makes a valuable contribution to the lives of people with disabilities. But as a medicalized form of normalizing therapy, it is subject to the more general critique of the medical model undertaken throughout Disability Studies, and to specific questions about its therapeutic efficacy.[16]

Whatever the successes of music therapy, the following discussion approaches disability and music from a decidedly different direction. Instead of using music as a therapeutic intervention aimed at normalization and possible cure, I will attend to the ways in which people with disabilities listen to music, specifically to the ways in which the experience of inhabiting an extraordinary body can inflect the perception and cognition of music. As discussed in chapter 6, experientialist philosophers, most notably George Lakoff and Mark Johnson, have persuaded us that we use our direct, concrete, physical knowledge of our own bodies as a basis for understanding the world around us: our knowledge of the world is embodied. Bodies therefore matter a great deal. But the bodies that Lakoff and Johnson have in mind are normal, standard bodies, unmarked by any differences or individuality, bodies that are, in fact, strangely abstract and disembodied. The experientialists blithely assume that

---

13. For an account of eighteenth-century descriptions of music as potentially either therapeutic or damaging, see LeGuin (2006). For a broader historical and cross-cultural perspective on the same topic, see Horden (2000).

14. As Hurt-Thaut (2009, 503) contends: "Music therapy is a health care profession in which music is used as a therapeutic medium to address developments, adaptive, and rehabilitative goals in the areas of psychosocial, cognitive, and sensorimotor behavior of individuals with disabilities."

15. For a characteristic example of the medical model of disability operating in music therapy, see Alvin and Warwick (1991), in which the music therapists are depicted as heroic figures offering the possibility of cure to their afflicted patients.

16. It is difficult to gauge the success of the music-therapeutic enterprise. McFerran et al. (2009) assesses the effectiveness of music therapy for people with disabilities (mostly children with intellectual, developmental, or cognitive impairments) by reviewing recent literature. The authors conclude that "music plays a powerful role in facilitating communication with this group of people and also providing a highly motivating context in which to establish relationships and maintain physical and behavioral achievements" (65). The actual, documented successes seem rather modest, however.

all people inhabit the same kind of body—a normatively abled body—and that all people thus experience their bodies in pretty much the same way.

This false, damaging assumption is reflected in their obsessive use of the first person plural: *our* reality, *our* bodily movement, *our* experiences, *our* bodies. One sees the same rhetorical power-grab throughout the literature on music cognition, in which the first person plural and the definite article exert a coercive force: *the* musical mind, *our* intuitions. As Lerdahl and Jackendoff (1983, 281) assert, "Much of the complexity of musical intuition is not learned, but is given by the inherent organization of the mind, itself determined by the human genetic inheritance."

To the contrary, differences in human embodiment—physical, psychological, cognitive, and intellectual differences—play a significant role in the ways people make sense of their world, including their musical world. Our bodies and minds are not all the same, and the differences among us make a difference.[17] If our goal is to understand how people make sense of music, we will have to accept that people vary in significant ways and that the senses they make of music will vary accordingly. It is as wrong to exclude from our studies of musical cognition people with physical, cognitive, and psychological differences as it would be to exclude people based on ethnicity or gender. People with disabilities are part of the human community, and if we want to know how people understand music, then we must include them as a matter equally of obtaining a full, accurate picture and of simple justice.[18]

Doubtless bringing people with disabilities to the center of our discussion of music cognition will complicate our studies and produce messier results, and that is

17. A critique of experientialism along these lines has appeared occasionally in the disability literature. See, for example, Dolmage (2005, 116): "When a different body conceptualizes the world, the world opens up and the fences come down." Likewise, Scully (2008) argues that phenomenologist and experientialist philosophers, like cognitive and neuroscientists, make a serious error in failing to take sufficient account of variation in bodies and their functioning, and the impact of that variation on cognition:

> From the perspective of disability, the truly striking thing about both phenomenological and neuroscientific theories is the virtually exclusive focus on normative forms of embodiment....Cognitive scientists, like most phenomenologists, have not yet acknowledged that the body of their subject does not necessarily adhere to a universal human form....I am not aware of any studies carried out with the embodied cognition paradigm that have tried specifically to take into account differences in perceptual and motor experiences that follow from having a body that senses or moves in a different way from the norm. This is a significant gap since, according to the embodied mind paradigm, it's the *particularities* of an organism's embodiment that largely determine the nature of the experiences that serve as a basis for cognition (94–95).

18. As Judith Butler (1999, 110) observes with regard to sexuality:

> The point here is not to seek recourse to the exceptions, the bizarre, in order merely to relativize the claims made in behalf of normal sexual life....It is the exception, the strange, that gives us the clue to how the mundane and taken-for-granted world of sexual meanings is constituted. Only from a self-consciously denaturalized position can we see how the appearance of naturalness is itself constituted....Hence, the strange, the incoherent, that which falls "outside," gives us a way of understanding the taken-for-granted world as a constructed one, as one that might well be constructed differently.

all to the good, as far as I am concerned. As Siebers (2008) observes, the same is true when people with disabilities are brought into any endeavor:

> When a disabled body enters any construction, social or physical, a deconstruction occurs, a deconstruction that reveals the lines of force, the blueprint, of the social rendering of the building as surely as its physical rendering. Constructions are built with certain social bodies in mind, and when a different body appears, the lack of fit reveals the ideology of ability controlling the space (124).

By deconstructing music cognition's unreflecting reliance on normal hearing, we can construct a new understanding of the ways people make sense of music as complex, varied, and diverse as people themselves.

Normal hearing is the way in which normally embodied people make sense of music. I would like to counterpoise this with what I will call "disablist hearing," that is, the ways in which people with disabilities make sense of music. In what follows, I consider four kinds of disablist hearing: autistic hearing, blind hearing, deaf hearing, and mobility-inflected hearing. Before getting into the details, however, it is necessary to confront and refute any charge of essentialism. I am not suggesting that all autistic, blind, deaf people, or people with mobility issues hear in the ways I describe, and I am not suggesting that to hear in these ways one needs to be autistic, blind, deaf, or mobility impaired. Like disability itself, hearing is a kind of performance—one may choose to hear normally and one may choose to hear in a disablist mode. My goal is not so much to classify ways of hearing as either normal or disablist, but rather to expand the range of hearings available to all of us, normatively embodied or not.

Because musical hearing is learned, not given, in principle all sorts of musical hearing are accessible to everyone. But in practice, for any of the modes of hearing described here, some effort may be required—sometimes considerable effort—and success is not guaranteed in advance. All modes of hearing involve a process of acculturation, which may include formal training. Some listeners may be more inclined, or better suited, for some modes than others. Prodigious listeners, with extraordinary musical skills, will have the easiest access to prodigious hearing. Likewise, listeners with certain disabilities may have easier access to certain kinds of disablist hearing. It is still true, however, that with appropriate training and effort, people with disabilities can hear normally, even prodigiously, and that nondisabled people can cultivate disablist hearing. That raises the attractive possibility of an ultimate deconstruction of the well-defended border between normal and disablist hearing.

AUTISTIC HEARING

Most discussions of autism take place within a medical model that defines it as a pathology. For example, the description of autism in the *Diagnostic and Statistical*

Manual of Mental Disorders (DSM)—the authoritative manual of psychiatric diagnoses—describes autism as involving impairments in social interaction and communication together with abnormally restricted or repetitive behaviors.[19] As with all psychiatric disorders, autism is defined as an insufficiency (or excess) with respect to an untheorized and undefined normal.

Recently, a nonmedical counternarrative has arisen within which autism is described as a cognitive and behavioral difference, not a deficit. This counternarrative has its roots in the Disability Rights movement and, specifically, in the movement toward "neurodiversity." In this view, autism is a way of being in the world, that is, a worldview; it is a difference, not a deficit. People writing from this point of view, including many individuals who are themselves on the autism spectrum, have identified a number of components to what they think of as an autistic "cognitive style." I will review three salient features of that style, which I will refer to as "local coherence," "private association," and "imitation." All three are widely described both in the medical/psychiatric literature as well as in the recent profusion of memoirs and other first-person accounts by individuals on the autism spectrum. For each of these attributes of autistic cognitive style, I will discuss how it might shape a disablist musical hearing.[20]

One prevalent theory of autism considers it a disorder characterized by "weak central coherence"—an atypically weak tendency to bind local details into global wholes.[21] In this view, the deficits in social relatedness, considered one of the three defining characteristics of autism in the DSM, as well as other intellectual deficits associated with autism, are manifestations of an underlying inability to create larger meanings or patterns from discrete elements.[22]

19. The history of autism diagnoses is traced in Grinker (2007). For a vigorous critique of the DSM as more a pragmatic, social document than a scientific one—it functions primarily to provide stable, consistently identifiable populations for researchers to study, drug companies to medicate, and insurance companies to reimburse—see Kutchins and Kirk (1997) and Lewis (2006). On autism as a cultural practice rather than a medical diagnosis, see Straus (2010). On the cultural basis of mental illness generally, see Watters (2010).

20. The discussion that follows is indebted to Headlam (2006), both for the general idea of "autistic hearing" and some of its specifics.

21. See Frith and Happé (1999) and Frith (2003). Like the "theory of mind" and "executive function" theories discussed below, the "weak central coherence" theory remains controversial due to its lack of demonstrable neurological or biological basis (see Schreibman 2005).

22. According to Frith (2003, 160),

> We have now enough evidence to formulate a hypothesis about the nature of the intellectual dysfunction in autism. In the normal cognitive system there is a built-in propensity to form coherence over as wide a range of stimuli as possible, and to generalize over as wide a range of contexts as possible. It is this drive that results in grand systems of thought, and it is this capacity for coherence that is diminished in children with autism. As a result, their information-processing systems, like their very beings, are characterized by detachment. Detachment, as a technical term, refers to a quality of thought. It could be due either to a lack of global coherence or to a resistance to such coherence.

To recast the same notion as a cognitive difference rather than a deficit, we might say that people with autism are often richly attentive to minute details. They have an unusual and distinctive ability to attend to details on their own terms, not subsumed into a larger totality. Objects are apprehended in their full discrete and concrete individuality rather than as members or representatives of a larger subsuming abstract category. Autistic cognition involves "detail-focused processing" (Happé 2005, 640); it is based on *local coherence*. [23]

Writing as an insider, a person with autism, Temple Grandin confirms this sense of details perceived in their full individuality without regard to a subsuming context or category:

> Unlike those of most people, my thoughts move from video-like, specific images to generalization and concepts. For example, my concept of dogs is inextricably linked to every dog I've ever known. It's as if I have a card catalogue of dogs I have seen, complete with pictures, which continually grows as I add more examples to my video library.... My memories usually appear in my imagination in strict chronological order, and the images I visualize are always specific. There is no generic, generalized Great Dane (Grandin 1995, 27–28).

How might this cognitive style based on local coherence play out in music? In the domain of pitch perception, absolute pitch (AP) is significantly more prevalent among people with autism than in the general population. As a nonrelational strategy of pitch perception, one based on the internal qualities of a tone without respect to other tones, AP would seem to epitomize an autistic cognition of music, based on local rather than central coherence. [24] More generally, we might speculate that, if normal listening emphasizes contextualization and patterning, autistic

---

23. For more on the recasting of "weak central coherence" (a deficit) as "local coherence" (a characteristic difference), see Mills (2008) and Belmonte (2008).

24. Absolute pitch is the ability to name a pitch or produce a pitch identified by name without using an external source. For a survey of work on absolute pitch, including the autism connection, see Ward (1999). Mottron et al. (1999, 486) suggests "a causal relationship between AP and autism," which they relate to an "atypical tendency to focus on the stimulus rather than its context." See also Brown et al. (2003, 166):

> Reports of a relatively high prevalence of absolute pitch (AP) in autistic disorder suggest that AP is associated with some of the distinctive cognitive and social characteristics seen in autism spectrum disorders.... Piecemeal information processing, of which AP is an extreme and rare example, is characteristic of autism and may be associated as well with subclinical variants in language and behavior. We speculate that the gene or genes that underlie AP may be among the genes that contribute to autism.... Inasmuch as AP possessors can identify the individual pitches in a melody, AP is an extreme example of piecemeal information processing.... The link between autism and AP points to other neuropsychological processes that might underlie AP. A number of the special abilities found in autistic savants—prodigious memory and AP among them—can be characterized as high-fidelity information processing...."

listening emphasizes the integrity of the discrete event, an orientation toward the part rather then the whole.

A second prevalent theory of autism contends that the central deficit is a lack of a "theory of mind": people with autism are deficient in the ability to attribute intentions, knowledge, and feelings to other people (Frith 2003; Baron-Cohen 1993, 1997, 2001, 2004).[25] As a result, people with autism have difficulties both with social relatedness and with communication (two of the three principal marks of autism, according to the DSM). Limitations in social relatedness and communication create the impression of isolation, as though the person with autism were living in a separate, self-enclosed world.[26] This notion underpins the label "autism" itself and resonates with Leo Kanner's contention that "aloneness" is one of the two defining features of autism ("sameness" is the other).[27]

Recent literature from inside the autism community recasts these apparent deficits as differences characteristic of a distinctively autistic cognitive style. In this alternative view, autistic thinking is based on locally coherent networks of private associations. Like poetry, especially modernist poetry, autistic language often involves unusual, idiosyncratic combinations of elements and images, with as much pleasure associated with the sounds of the words as with their meaning. In Kristina Chew's (2008, 142, 133) words,

> Autistic language is a fractioned idiom, its vocabulary created from contextual and seemingly arbitrary associations of word and thing, and peculiar to its sole speaker alone.... Autistic language users think metonymically, connecting and ordering concepts according to seemingly chance and arbitrary occurrences in an "autistic idiolect."[28]

25. The questionable term "mindblindness" is sometimes used with reference to this cognitive deficit. The concept of the "theory of mind" has encountered significant resistance in the literature. For a discussion of the absence of a biological basis, see Schreibman (2005). For its refutation by the presence of numerous first-person accounts by autistic authors, replete with representations of their own mental states and the mental states of others, see McGeer (2004). For a critique from within the autism community, see Nazeer (2006, 68–75).

26. Metaphors that emphasize the separation of two worlds—a private, inner autistic world and a public, outer, normal social world, with the boundary between the two often figured as a wall—are extremely common in the professional literature and parent memoirs. They are rare, however, in the first-person literature.

27. Kanner coined the term "autism" and provided the first systematic description of it. The conceptual framework he established still shapes contemporary understanding of autism. See Kanner (1943, 1949).

28. Roman Jakobson's well-known discussion of "The Metaphoric and Metonymic Poles" (Jakobson 1971) is relevant here. For Jakobson, the "metonymic way" is bound up with combination and contiguity: events or images are brought into relationship with each other based on their association and proximity. In contrast, the "metaphoric way" is bound up with similarity and substitution: events or images are brought into relationship with each other based on their shared qualities, making it possible for one to stand for the other.

Temple Grandin (1975, 173) expresses the same notion in personal terms:

> One of my students remarked that horses don't think, they must make associations. If making associations is not considered thought, then I would have to conclude that I am unable to think. Thinking in visual pictures and making associations is simply a different form of thinking from verbal-based linear thought. There are advantages and disadvantages to both kinds of thinking. Ask any artist or accountant.

In relation to the perception and cognition of music, we should imagine an autistic listener as someone more attuned to private, idiosyncratic associations than larger shared meanings. Autistic hearing is both private and "fractionated." If normal hearing involves the creation of hierarchies, locally coherent autistic hearing involves a refusal to subsume perceptions into a hierarchy—individual events are full and complete in themselves, not operating the service of a higher totality (Headlam 2006). Instead of hierarchy, autistic hearing involves the creation of associative networks.[29] Individual events are not so much clumped together to create larger patterns as they are appreciated both for their own sake and for the associations they may evoke in relation to other individual events.

A third prevalent theory of autism relates autistic behavior to deficiencies in the brain's "executive function." People with autism often manifest "restricted, repetitive, and stereotyped patterns of behavior, interests, and activities" (DSM), which, according to this theory, result from difficulties in modulating mental focus, or shifting attention easily from task to task. This resonates with Kanner's second principal defining feature of autism, namely its insistence on "sameness."

Of course obsession and single-mindedness can be highly desirable traits—artistic creativity, for example, depends upon them. Autistic fixity of focus is a quality that enables another characteristic of autistic cognition, what Oliver Sacks refers to as a "gift for mimesis" (Sacks 1995, 241). People with autism, especially those with so-called "savant skills," often have prodigious rote memories.[30] In relation to music

29. As autistic author Gunilla Gerland (1997, 65–66) observes,

> There was something special about the way I saw things. My vision was rather flat, two-dimensional in a way, and this was somehow important to the way I viewed space and people. I seemed to have to fetch visual impressions from my eyes. Visual impressions did not come to *me*. Nor did my vision provide me with any automatic priority in what I saw—everything seemed to appear just as clearly and with the same sharpness of image. The world looked like a photograph.

30. The literature on musical memory in people with autism, often referred to in the past with the offensive label "idiot savant," includes Révész (1925), Hermelin et al. (1987), Miller (1987, 1989), Treffert (1988), Sloboda (2005), and Ockelford (2007). Although the offensiveness of the first word in that earlier label is clear enough, the term "savant" is also problematic. First, it entails an invidious comparison between the narrow ability (the "splinter skill") and the larger disability. Instead it might be better to see the variety of skills possessed by an individual person in the same way we see the variety of skills possessed by groups of people, as aspects of naturally occurring and desirable diversity. Second, it carries an impulse

perception and cognition, we should imagine an autistic listener as someone with a preference for repetition and with the cognitive capacity for recalling extended musical passages in full detail. Like absolute pitch, prodigious rote memory epitomizes autistic hearing. And, in this sense at least, autistic hearing may also be prodigious hearing.

In the portrait I have painted here, an autistic listener is someone who attends to the discrete musical event in all of its concrete detail (local coherence); who prefers the part to the whole; who is adept at creating associative networks (often involving private or idiosyncratic meanings); and who may have absolute pitch and a prodigious rote memory. To these three features of autistic hearing, I would like to add one more: people with autism sometimes respond to music with their own vocalizations—they experience music in part through singing or humming, and the sounds they make function as a mode of apprehension.[31] Among musical performers with autism, we have already noted in chapter 7 the extensive vocalizations of "Blind Tom" and Glenn Gould—these were apparently indispensable parts of their way of making music.[32]

In each of these respects, autistic hearing provides an alternative to normal hearing, which is undertaken in silence and oriented toward global coherence, the synthesis of wholes from parts, the creation of relationships among discrete events, the subsuming context, and the creation of conceptual hierarchies, particularly in the domain of pitch. As noted earlier, I am not suggesting that all people with autism hear autistically, or that you have to be autistic to hear autistically. Rather, autistic hearing is a mode of hearing associated with autism.

Normal hearing is well suited to the traditional tonal repertoire. This is the music that cognitive scientists have mostly focused on and on which they have based their conclusions about human cognition. In listening to traditional tonal music, many listeners use cognitive strategies based on the creation of pitch hierarchies. But it would be wrong to conclude either that these strategies are the only way to listen to tonal music, or (even more damagingly) that only music that rewards such strategies can be good music. On the first point, alternative ways of hearing, ways that have strong affinities with autistic hearing with its emphasis on local networks of associations, can also be rewarding and revealing for traditional tonal music.[33] You

---

toward "enfreakment": the special skill provokes amazement and wonder, and also a sense of irreducible otherness (the skill seems almost inhuman). Third, the "autistic savant" comes to play the same role with respect to the population of autistic people that the "supercrip" does with respect to disabled people; it minimizes the challenges that most people with disabilities face and implies an additional burden, possibly a moral burden, of failing to measure up to an unrealistic standard.

31. I credit this observation to Stephanie Jensen-Moulton (private communication).

32. See Malone (2000) for fascinating transcriptions and analyses of Gould's vocalizations.

33. This is a central contention of Boros (1995). Ashby (2004, 33–35) argues along similar lines:

do not have to hear normally (i.e., hierarchically) to make enjoyable sense of traditional tonal music.

On the second point, modernist atonal music may simultaneously discourage normal hearing and encourage autistic hearing. As Amy Bauer (2004, 124) observes,

> Lerdahl and Rochberg's theories tacitly present tonal and other hierarchically structured musics as metaphoric models of "normal" cognition, with the implication that atonal and other non-hierarchically structured musics model "abnormal" states of mind. In effect, cognitive constraints function less as a *requirement for,* than a *description of,* ordinary cognition. If modern music lacks all the elements necessary for comprehensibility, then it must describe an altered state of cognition, perhaps even psychosis. Music that flouts cognitive constraints might even represent a kind of reified madness.[34]

If normal hearing is not suitable for atonal music, it does not follow that atonal music cannot be good music. Instead, we need to engage different strategies of

---

> I don't believe music, even serial music, need be limited to a grammatical-linguistic conception of meaning. I would go further and say that modern art—or art in any period, for that matter—need not function grammatically.... One could fault Lerdahl for failing to differentiate between things one *could* follow [i.e., serial things] and things an auditor *should* or likely *does* follow, and for implying that it is the former that tells us which listener will "understand" which compositions. I don't believe most listeners hear many tonal details that are essential to the compositional structure of works from the common practice period, but that doesn't invalidate those structures and relations.

Likewise, Dubiel (2008) states: "Let me propose to value the formation of hierarchies not as a necessity, but as an option and even as an extravagance. And let the ability to find one's way around without a strict system, and to deal with multiplicity, be recognized as a mental ability at least as valuable." Likewise, Smith (2006, 146–47) emphasizes that important features of traditional tonal music may be cognized nonhierarchically:

> One of the chief advantages of a Schenkerian approach is its ability to respond to functional distinctions among tonal events that only incidentally possess the same chord grammar. A healthy trend in recent years, however, has been a counterbalancing recognition of the limits of this kind of hierarchical hearing in responding to aspects of coherence in works of the great tonal tradition.

Cook (1994) summarizes studies of tonal music and concludes that listeners do not generally listen grammatically (hierarchically); rather, they listen for salience, just as they do for atonal music: "If people (musically trained people) listen to tonal and atonal music in much the same way, and if atonal music is not very grammatical, then tonal music cannot be very grammatical either" (72).

34. In less charged language, Morris (1995, 356) also argues for the primacy of association rather than hierarchy in atonal music:

> If spaces are not musical grammars, they substitute for such grammars by using association rather than chunking as their underlying psycho-cognitive mechanism. This reflects the fact that today's music need not be primarily hierarchic in order to have the richness of affiliation and scope of reference so often associated with the tonal music of earlier musical periods.

listening—perhaps we need to learn to hear autistically.[35] Atonal music thus appears as a built environment that disables normal listeners while enabling disablist listeners.

DEAF HEARING

At first blush, "deaf hearing" seems like an oxymoron. The prevalent view of deafness is that it involves an absolute inability to hear, a life of total silence.[36] But this is mostly false. The large majority of people classified as deaf, and most people who identify themselves as Deaf, have some degree of hearing. As Padden and Humphries (1988, 93) observe,

> When hearing people identify Deaf people as silent, they are mistakenly assuming that Deaf people have no concept of sound, that sound plays no part in their world, or that if it does, their ideas about it are deeply distorted. The truth is that many Deaf people know a great deal about sound, and that sound itself—not just its absence—plays a central role in their lives.

What is most distinctive about deaf hearing, however, is the extent to which deaf people use senses other than the auditory to make sense of what they hear: they see and feel music. Hearing does not necessarily involve a one-to-one mapping of sense perceptions onto a single sensory organ; rather, hearing can be a much more multisensory experience.

The visual plays a central role in Deaf culture.[37] George Veditz, a president of the National Association of the Deaf, famously observed in 1910 that deaf people were

35. This conclusion tracks a central argument in Headlam (2006).
36. The visual counterpart of deaf hearing would be blind seeing, an interesting area of study, although beyond the scope of this book. This issue is discussed extensively in Kleege (1999). See also Davidson (2008), which includes a discussion of blind photographers such as Alice Wingwall, Evgen Bavcar, and Derek Jarman in a chapter titled "Nostalgia for Light: Being Blind at the Museum," and makes reference to a conference at the University of California-Berkeley Art Museum called "Blind at the Museum" (2005). In a related vein, Deaf artist and philosopher Joseph Grigely (2000) refers to "the tactile gaze of the blind": "This touching is not about feeling, not about touching even, but about seeing. Touching itself is elided; it is a semantic projection of our own physiology, not that of the blind. If everyone in the world were blind, perhaps touching would be called seeing" (33).
37. As Bauman (2008, 1, 9) shows,

> Among the seismic shifts in culture brought about in the 1960s was a much quieter but nonetheless profound revolution in our understanding of human language and culture: the validation of the fully linguistic nature of sign languages and the subsequent rewriting of deaf identity from deaf to Deaf, that is, from a pathological state of hearing loss to the cultural identity of a linguistic minority.... Rewriting deaf to Deaf is about disowning an imposed medicalized identity and developing an empowered identity rooted in a community and culture of others who share similar experiences and outlooks on the world.

"first and foremost and for all time, people of the eye" (Veditz 1912, 30, cited in Bauman 2008, 12).[38] In Benjamin Bahan's phrase, deaf people are "a visual variety of the human race" (Bahan 2008). In Tobin Siebers's (2008, 53) poetic formulation: "All disabled bodies create [a] confusion of tongues—and eyes and hands and other body parts. For the deaf, the hand is the mouth of speech, the eye, its ear. Deaf hands speak. Deaf eyes listen."

The visual features of music are generally ignored in studies of music cognition, where the listener is imagined as someone alone in a room listening to recorded sounds. But, of course, a much more common context for hearing music involves the eyes as well as the ears—we see music being made, or we see ourselves making music. A visual listener will be attuned to musical features that might otherwise be ignored by nonvisual listeners. A visual listener—and deaf people are primarily visual listeners—will hear and understand music differently.

Here is an illustrative example. Studies in music cognition have been interested in the perception of key—they want to know how listeners ascertain musical key and to what extent they are aware of changes in key, including a final return to the tonic key. In general, listeners (normal, nonvisual listeners) are not very good at apprehending large-scale tonal relations (Cook 1987). But this task becomes considerably easier if the listener can see the performers. If you can see an instrument being played, and you have some basic idea about how instruments produce pitch (e.g., the lowest string on the cello is a C), it is relatively easy to know what key the music is in at any point. A key, in other words, can be seen as well as heard. Not only will visual listeners (deaf listeners) be better than normal listeners at apprehending large-scale key relations, so will absolute-pitch listeners (autistic listeners). This is an important, higher-level cognitive task of the kind that is most highly valued by traditional tonal theory, and it is one on which deaf and autistic listeners, like Schenker's prodigious listeners, perform better than normal listeners.

Deaf hearing involves the tactile as well as the visual. Bauman describes the Deaf as "visual-tactile minority living in a phonocentric world" (Bauman 2008, 4). As Padden and Humphries (1988, 94) observe, "For many deaf people, the lower frequencies are the most easily detectable, creating not only loud sounds they can hear but vibrations on the floor and furniture." Within the Deaf cultural world, music is often projected so as to maximize its felt vibrations (audio speakers placed face down on the ground, so that vibrations can be felt by dancing feet, or balloons held in hands to enhance sonic vibration).

Deaf musical hearing thus involves not only seeing music but feeling it as well. The idea of tactile hearing is beautifully expressed by the deaf percussionist

38. Translated slightly differently in Bahan (2008, 83): "[Deaf people] are first, last and of all time the people of the eye." Yet another translation is offered in Baynton (2008, 293): "[Deaf people] are first, last and all the time *the* people of the eye." I would guess that these discrepancies result from different translations of a speech given in American Sign Language (ASL).

Evelyn Glennie, whose approach to music-making was a subject of chapter 7. She argues that "hearing is basically a specialized form of touch" (Glennie 2010a) and that "I can also tell the quality of a note by what I feel, I can sense musical sound through my feet and lower body, and also through my hands; and can identify the different notes as I press the pedal according to which part of my foot feels the vibrations and for how long, and by how I experience the vibrations in my body" (Glennie 1990, 73). Deaf hearing thus involves sensory input from a variety of sources—it is not confined to the ears.[39]

Hearing music by feeling it may extend beyond the tactile to the kinesthetic.[40] One can hear music, make sense of music, cognize music, by moving or dancing to it. As Neumeyer (2006) points out, a listener who is also a dancer may experience and understand music differently from the immobile, passive listener of the psychological studies.[41] Specifically, a listener who is also a dancer is likely to be more attuned to musical rhythm than the normal listener. Let us then imagine a deaf listener as one who engages the visual, the tactile, and the kinesthetic in apprehending music: deaf hearing involves seeing, feeling, and moving to music.[42] Of course deaf listeners can learn to hear "normally," and hearing listeners can learn deaf hearing; these are modes of apprehension, not essential attributes of bodies.

Deaf hearing may also be silent and inward. Inner hearing—the ability to conceptualize music in its full particularity in the absence of audible sound—is a

39. A recent comment by H-Dirksen Bauman nicely expresses this multisensory understanding of hearing. He argues that,

> The traditional parsing of senses in the West is a bit of a folk belief that links each sense with a particular organ, instead of seeing perception as a more malleable, synesthetic process. Given our focus on the ways that Deaf ways of being bring about an alternative alignment of sensory perception, the role of alternative hearing has often come up in our discussions. As a means of expressing this, we use the handshape for the sign to "hear" and place it on the hands, or arm, or chest, to signify the ways that the skin and muscle "hear" "sound" (private communication, June 13, 2008).

40. For interesting studies of the "cross-modal" relationship between sound and visual or kinesthetic imagery, see Eitan and Granot (2006) and Eitan and Timmers (2010).

41. The kinesthetics of performance may also affect cognition, as Quinn observes. In reference to a claim in Lerdahl (1988) that "the best music utilizes the full potential of our cognitive resources," Quinn (2006, 293) observes that "performance can easily stretch the limits of cognitive resources." In other words, the listener who is also a performer understands music differently.

42. In the succinct formulation of an accomplished deaf musician, Tammie Willis, "the meaning I derive from my perceptions is really based on three components, what I feel, what I see, and what I know" (private communication). Although my focus here is on deaf listeners and deaf hearing, an important related topic is deaf music-making. Prominent here are two forms of ASL (American Sign Language) songs. In the first, ASL is presented as a form of translation and interpretation of an existing song, as a visual and rhythmic counterpoint (Bahan [2006] calls these "translated songs"). In the second, an idiomatic "visual-sound music" is composed directly in ASL. One form of these are what Bahan calls "percussion signing," which involves arranging signs into rhythmic patterns. These latter are part of what Bahan refers to as "the face-to-face tradition" in deaf culture, a tradition that includes storytelling, poetry, and forms of visual music.

distinguishing ability of trained musicians and a central focus of musical education. It is obviously a crucial ability for performers (who need to know, silently and in advance, what sound they are to produce) and composers.[43] It is also characteristic of a certain mode of contemplative hearing in which music, in either the presence or absence of musical notation, is perceived and understood in the musical mind.[44] One advantage to such silent hearing is the freedom from the constraint of time— one can move backward as well as forward in a work, dwelling on particular details, attending to particular relationships, freely and at will. Deaf hearing may thus also be hearing out of time. One aspect of this out-of-time way of hearing may be a reliance on visual imagery or models; even "hearing" listeners, when they want to think about structural features, often turn to visual and spatial models.[45] In all of these respects—hearing as seeing, hearing as feeling, hearing as movement, hearing as silent, out-of-time contemplation—deaf hearing provides an alternative to normal hearing.

BLIND HEARING

If "deaf hearing" sounds like an oxymoron, "blind hearing" may sound like a tautology: in the popular imagination, blind people are compensated for their disability with preternaturally acute hearing as well as prodigious musical gifts. It is certainly true that many blind people have learned to be extremely sensitive, acute listeners (just as many deaf people have learned to be extremely sensitive, acute visual observers).[46] In fact, however, blind people are innately no more musically gifted

43. Glennie (1990, 72) asserts that she accesses music via notation and inner hearing, not by listening to other people play: "I didn't need to listen to music because I could read it like a book."

44. As Sacks (2007, 33–34) observes,

> Deliberate, conscious, voluntary mental imagery involves not only the auditory and motor cortex, but regions of the frontal cortex involved in choosing and planning. Such deliberate mental imagery is clearly crucial to professional musicians—it saved the creative life and sanity of Beethoven after he had gone deaf and could no longer hear any music other than that in his mind. (It is possible, indeed, that his musical imagery was even intensified by deafness, for with the removal of normal auditory input, the auditory cortex may become hypersensitive, with heightened powers of musical imagery.)

45. See Hook (2002, 123), with the apt title "Hearing with our Eyes." Hook argues,

> Most human beings are visually oriented. We rely on our eyes more than our ears or any of our other sense organs in finding our way around, identifying other people and objects, and learning new information. Because of this dependence on the visual world, most people find abstract concepts easier to grasp if they can somehow be *visualized*: if some sort of graphical, geometric representation can be devised showing, if only metaphorically, the important elements of the conceptual framework and their relationships with each other. Even if these elements exist in sound and time rather than in light and space, such a representation may help us to get our bearings and to interpret what we hear.

46. As Kuusisto (2006, xi) observes,

than sighted people.[47] At the same time, as discussed in chapter 1, blind people are often tracked into musical activities, and there is a long history of distinguished blind musicians in all times and places.

The number and variety of blind musicians make it difficult to generalize about blind hearing (the same is true even of the smaller number of autistic, deaf, and mobility-impaired musicians). One shared feature, however, is that for blind musicians, and blind listeners generally, the experience of music is usually not mediated by notation. When we study the cognition of experienced, classically trained musicians, we are studying a class of people who come to music through its notation. As composers, we notate our musical ideas, and those ideas are shaped by our ability to write them down. As performers, we learn to play our part by reading it in notation, and even after we set the notation aside, we may conjure it up in our visual memory as we play. As listeners, if we have sufficient musical training, we may create notation in our musical minds as we listen—the heard sounds leave a visual trace in the form of imagined, recreated musical notation. The term musicians use for reading music notation and making aural sense of it is "sight singing," which suggests the centrality for musical understanding of music notation *as seen*.[48] For experienced, classically trained musicians, then, notation-based hearing is normal hearing.[49]

Blind hearing, on the other hand, is unmediated by notation. If we think about music globally—including non-Western and popular music—we realize that notation-based hearing (or music-making generally) is very much the minority. What I am calling blind hearing is statistically far more common than notation-based hearing. Blind hearing, as I imagine it, may be more sensitive to aspects of music

---

Blindness often leads to compensatory listening....I used the term "compensatory listening" just now but I could substitute "creative listening." Blind people are not casual eavesdroppers. We have methods. As things happen around us we reinvent what we hear like courtroom artists who sketch as fast as they can.... In reality I cannot see the world by ear, I can only reinvent it for my own purposes.

See also Kleege (1999).

47. There is some evidence, however, that absolute pitch (AP) is more prevalent among people with visual impairments than within the general population. See Hamilton et al. (2004), Pring et al. (2008), and Gaab et al. (2006). According to Sacks (2007, 126), "There is a striking association of absolute pitch with early blindness (some studies estimate that about 50 percent of children born blind or blinded in infancy have absolute pitch)."

48. As Lerner and Straus (2006, 1) observe,

The language musicians use says much about their assumptions. For example, *sight singing* constitutes a basic element in music education. To perform music within the cultivated tradition, musicians are expected to read musical notation, and so the study of sight singing cultivates the skill of translating printed musical notation into performed sound. Yet the implication behind the phrase sight singing assumes something more: that one must have sight to read music.

49. In the field of music psychology, there is a small literature on the acquisition of the skill of reading music notation (see Sloboda [2005], for example). But I am not aware of any attempt to study the impact of the ability to read music notation on the cognition of music.

that are not conveyed by traditional musical notation, aspects that Hatten (2004, 199) refers to as "microstructures": "variables in sound production that fall between the cracks of our discrete notational system." Blind hearing might thus be more sensitive than normal, notation-based hearing to shifts in such things as articulation, dynamics, tuning, or timbre.[50]

In the domain of pitch, blind hearing may be less subject than normal hearing to what Westergaard (1996, 18) refers to as "the diatonic bias of the staff." As Westergaard poetically observes, traditional notation is not neutral—it tells us how to hear and, given the history and structure of traditional staff notation, it tells us to hear in terms of diatonic scales:

> I think we all too often tacitly
> assume that our notation's just a set
> of orders telling someone else what he
> or she must do with hands or throat to get
> the sounds required. There are notations that do
> just that, but ours does more, far more. It tells
> you how to think of the sounds you are to make (17).

Normal hearing, as constructed by studies in music cognition, is inflected by what Cook (1994, 81) calls "theorism": "the premise that people hear music in terms of music-theoretical categories. [Music psychologists] assume what music theory assumes, that music is made out of notes." Cook observes,

> If music theorists really wanted to analyze how music sounds, and only how it sounds, they would put away their scores and forget all about notes. Some phenomenologically minded theorists have tried to do just this. The trouble is that they almost invariably end up creating scores of their own. The only difference is that their scores tend to be relatively impoverished representations of the music, so the analytical results are generally unsatisfying from a musical point of view. This is not really surprising.... Music theorists can no more forget about notes than linguists can forget about letters; they are part of our mental equipment (80).

For Cook, then, normal hearing—in which listeners are assumed to be attentive to key relations and to be cognizing hierarchical pitch relationships in multiple structural levels—is more an artifact of notation-based studies than an accurate reflection of general music cognition. In this sense, Cook's theorism is what I am calling

---

50. For a discussion along similar lines, see LeGuin (2004). She documents her experience listening to a Debussy song—just listening to it, without score—and finds it is nearly impossible to process the music without thinking in terms of notation. She also finds her mind focusing on localized events, gestures, etc., at the expense of key relationships.

notation-based normal hearing, and Cook's listeners are like my blind listeners—relatively indifferent to the hierarchical pitch structures embodied in music notation and emphasized in studies of music cognition.

In the absence of traditional staff notation, perhaps blind hearing becomes more tactile, more grounded in the physical knowledge of an instrument. Musicians all hear, to some extent, via their embodied knowledge of playing an instrument. When hearing music, musicians often imagine how it would feel when played, using a mental representation based on touch and physical movement rather than notation. Although such a tactile way of hearing is widespread among musicians, it may be intensified among blind listeners, undistracted by the more abstract appeal of music notation. If that is true, then blind hearing and deaf hearing would share an orientation toward the tactile and the kinesthetic.

Although blind listeners approach music without the mediation of traditional music notation, some make use of Braille music notation.[51] Braille music notation uses the same six-position cell as literary Braille—cells are distinguished by different patterns of raised dots—but the complexities of music notation require separate cells for pitch, accidental (i.e., sharp, natural, or flat), octave position, duration, and articulation. What's important is not whether Braille notation or traditional notation is more efficient—they both have advantages and disadvantages—but rather the sorts of cognitive biases that are embedded in each.[52] Two relevant biases come to mind. First, although traditional notation cultivates a spatial sense of music (the position of a note on the staff corresponds to its register, higher or lower), Braille notation does not.[53] Braille

51. This tactile form of music notation was developed by Louis Braille and published along with his better-known literary code in 1829. For a description of Braille music notation and discussion of its impact on music perception and cognition, see Johnson (2009). There is evidence that Braille reading is becoming less prevalent among blind people, who are turning increasingly toward computer-based access to written materials (see Aviv 2010). I am not aware of documentation of any similar, or contrary, trend among users of Braille music notation.

52. One functional difference between standard and Braille notations is worth noting. Because Braille notation occupies the hands, it is generally not suitable for real-time musical performance. In contrast, traditional notation is designed to be read and performed *at sight* (an apt phrase that captures the inescapably visual aspect of traditional notation).

53. Johnson (2008) observes,

> Such assumptions extend even to the most basic of musical concepts. For example, musicians speak of high and low pitches more as a result of the orientation of notes on the printed page rather than, say, notes on the piano where higher is to the *right* of the keyboard, or on the cello, where higher notes are played by placing fingers *lower* on the fingerboard. Sighted musicians also use the orientation of notes on the printed page to regulate time: for example, vertically aligned notes occur simultaneously and notes that are closer together horizontally are played more quickly. Writers such as Lawrence Zbikowski, Jana Saslaw, Arnie Cox and others have written extensively on how we musicians make use of embodied notions called image schemas (like VERTICALITY for high and low pitches) to structure our ideas about music. Print notation shares much of that image-schematic structure, and thus acts as an iconic representation of audible music by providing symbols that share many visual properties with the musical features they represent.

See also Johnson (2009).

notation might thus serve to undermine certain widely shared metaphors for musical perception, including the idea that pitches are arrayed vertically from high to low. Would blind listeners who come to music through Braille notation be less inclined than normal listeners to hear pitches as relatively high or low? What metaphors would they be more likely to use, and what would the impact of these metaphors be on their perception of pitch? I am not aware of any research that bears on these questions, but just to pose them is to suggest the limitations of normal, notation-based hearing.

Second, although traditional notation conveys a sense of simultaneity—notes that sound at the same time are vertically aligned on the page—Braille notation is more oriented towards distinct contrapuntal strands: the music is presented one melodic line at a time. There is thus a kind of contrapuntal bias built into the notation. In both senses, Braille notation conveys a sense of music as more diffuse, less fully integrated within a single conceptual space. Would blind listeners who come to music through Braille notation be more oriented toward a counterpoint of individual lines and less oriented toward vertical, harmonic integration? Again, this is an open question, and answering it might serve to broaden our sense of what is natural and normal in human hearing.

Like the listener who comes to music without the mediation of any notational system, the listener who comes to music through Braille notation may have an orientation away from the regime of pitch-based and notation-based "theorism." If normal hearing is grounded in theoretical concepts associated with traditional notation—and certainly many of the psychological experiments that construct normal hearing require a knowledge and practice of traditional music notation—then blind hearing may provide a valuable alternative.[54]

MOBILITY-INFLECTED HEARING

How might a nonnormative way of moving through the world, either with a halting gait or with a wheelchair, affect perception and cognition, including the perception and cognition of music? Experientialists like Lakoff and Johnson (discussed in chapter 6), argue that our understanding of abstract concepts is grounded in our prior concrete experience of our own bodies, and that prominent among the universal bodily experiences are "balance" and "verticality."

> Balance is something we experience immediately with our bodies. It involves our felt sense of an upright posture in which forces acting on us are organized around a central axis so that we remain upright, relatively in control of our actions, able to function effectively, and feeling somewhat stable. We know the meaning of balance pre-reflectively, in

54. See, for example, Deliège (1987), in which subjects were supplied with simplified scores and asked to draw vertical lines to delineate phrases and other segments in music they were listening to.

and through our bodies, even without thinking about it or conceptualizing it. Notice that there is what we might call a corporeal logic of our bodily balance: being balanced permits you to function successfully to achieve your ends (Johnson 1997–98, 98).

The "verticality" schema is based on "our felt sense of standing upright... the vertical orientation of our bodies" (Zbikowski 1997–98, 6).

Balance and verticality are certainly widely shared experiences, but they are in no sense universal. There are plenty of people whose normal posture is not upright, balanced, and vertical. People who walk and people who use wheelchairs move through the world in different ways. These different experiences of motion—a jerky motion through a series of near falls versus a smooth glide— may lead to subtle shifts in perception and cognition. John Hockenberry gives an evocative description of the contrast, based on his experience as a former walker and later a wheelchair user who finds himself riding a donkey in war-torn Kurdistan:

> Neither the heroic foot-borne relief efforts, anticipation of the horrors ahead, nor the brilliance of the scenery around me struck home as much as the rhythm of the donkey's forelegs beneath my hips. It was walking, that feeling of groping and climbing and floating on stilts that I had not felt for fifteen years. It was a feeling no wheelchair could convey. I had long ago grown to love my own wheels and their special physical grace, and so this clumsy leg walk was not something I missed until the sensation came rushing back though my body from the shoulders of a donkey (Hockenberry 1995, 2–3).[55]

The brilliant young pianist Stefan Honisch suggests a number of ways in which his wheelchair use, coming after years of increasing difficulty walking, has shaped his musical perceptions and his musical performance. His remarks, offered before a concert of music by Bach, Beethoven, and Chopin, are evocative and worth quoting at some length:

> Each of the works which I will perform for you tonight has been part of two very different time-periods in my life, past and present: the period, long past, in which, as a high school student, and then an undergraduate, I was still walking, albeit with a noticeable lack of fluency, and the present, in which as a doctoral student, I use only a wheelchair to move through the world. My interpretive view of these works has changed considerably, not only as a result of further study, but also, it seems to me, as a result of my changed perspective of the world as seen from a wheelchair. I now experience musical time in these works as much smoother, much less laborious, characterized by a hitherto unfamiliar kind of momentum. I find that the sensation of "rolling" along the ground on wheels shapes the circular motions which my hands describe at the keyboard in the

55. For more on the contrast between walking and gliding through the world, see Mairs (1996), H. Johnson (2005), and Linton (2006).

search for a legato sound. The piano keyboard, my navigations over it, my experience of being more or less connected to it, are colored by my physical perception of being connected to the ground underneath my feet and wheels: increasingly, I find it easier to play staccato passages with my feet off the ground, and to execute legato phrases with my feet firmly planted on the floor underneath. My past recollections of the effort involved in walking shape my interpretation of the [Chopin] Fantasy in F minor: a teacher of mine suggested, vividly, that the opening "Alla Marcia" section should feel as though one is "over-coming" each beat. I have found a helpful point of correspondence between his metaphorical interpretation of this music, and my own experience of walking, in which each step felt like an act of "overcoming." The way I understand the concept of "tempo rubato" has also undergone a noticeable transformation. When I was still walking, my perception of motion as goal-directed was almost constantly undermined by the sheer effort of moving. In order simply to remain upright, I had to focus awareness on what I was doing, with a consequent ignorance of where I was starting and where I was going. This is analogous in musical performance to focusing so much attention on each beat, or each note within a phrase, and the muscular movements necessary for their execution that one ceases to think of the goal of a phrase, or a section of music, or of maintaining a coherent pace. The fluidity of movement in a wheelchair significantly informs my understanding of tempo rubato. Knowing that physical movement is not necessarily painfully laborious, I can draw on my embodied experience of flexible pacing in a wheelchair, to inform the ways in which I rhythmically inflect the music I perform. I have recently begun to question whether my experience of moving through the world in a wheelchair might somehow be at the core of my preference for matters of detail in musical interpretation. Does viewing the world from the ground up, or more accurately, near the ground and looking up translate, musically, into an embodied inclination toward viewing works of music from a near-the-ground perspective, as opposed to a "bird's eye view" to invoke another common metaphorical formulation? This question remains unanswered for the present (Honisch 2010).

For Honisch, then, the embodied experience of moving through the world in a wheelchair shapes his music-making in a variety of ways, creating a sense of smooth motion through time, with more focus on long-range goals, and possibly greater attention to detail from a "near-the-ground perspective." We might speculate that wheelchair use might give rise to another sort of disablist hearing, one in which music tends to be perceived as a continuous flow, rather than a series of punctuated events (Honisch 2010).

ASSISTIVE TECHNOLOGIES, PROSTHESES, PERSONAL ASSISTANTS, AND THE MYTH OF AUTONOMY

Normal hearing involves a listener alone in a room, listening to recorded sounds: nothing to see, nothing to touch, no opportunity to move, no active participation (playing or singing), and above all, no intervention or assistance from anyone else. Normal listening is a solitary activity, something each person does alone in the privacy of his or her own individual, autonomous mind.

This prevalent idea of hearing as a solitary activity expresses deep-seated Western, and especially American, ideas of autonomy, individuality, independence, and self-sufficiency. As Martha Fineman (2004, 34) observes:

> American political ideology offers an iconic construct of the autonomous individual and trusts the abstraction of an efficiency-seeking market as an ordering mechanism. We have an historic and highly romanticized affair with the ideals of the private and the individual, as contrasted with the public and the collective, as the appropriate units of focus in determining social good.... Dependency is a particularly unappealing and stigmatized term in American political and popular consciousness. The specter of dependency is incompatible with our beliefs and myths. We venerate the autonomous, independent, and self-sufficient individual as our ideal. We assume that anyone can cultivate these characteristics, consistent with our belief in the inherent equality of all members of our society, and we stigmatize those who do not.

The Disability Rights movement, the field of Disability Studies, and the lived lives of people with disabilities all argue against the "myth of autonomy." In a world that includes personal assistants, classroom aides, service animals, sign-language interpreters, and visual describers, people with disabilities understand that they, and all of us, are sustained by and bound together in extensive webs of mutual dependence. As historian and activist Paul Longmore (2003, 222) notes,

> Some people with physical disabilities have been affirming the validity of values drawn from their own experience. Those values are markedly different from, and even opposed to, nondisabled majority values. They declare that they prize not self-sufficiency but self-determination, not independence but interdependence, not functional separateness but personal connection, not physical autonomy but human community. This values formation takes disability as the starting point. It uses the disability experience as the source of values and norms.[56]

56. Likewise, see Siebers (2008, 182):

> A focus on disability provides another perspective by representing human society not as a collection of autonomous beings, some of whom will lose their independence, but as a community of dependent frail bodies that rely on others for survival.... My point is not that disabled persons are dependent because of their individual properties or traits. It is not a matter of understanding disability as weakness but of construing disability as a critical concept that reveals the structure of dependence inherent to all human societies. As finite beings who live under conditions of scarcity, we depend on other human beings not only at those times when our capacities are diminished but each and every day, and even at those moments when we may be at the height of our physical and mental powers.

People with disabilities make use of assistance of all kinds to augment their powers and permit them to engage in a full range of activities. Sometimes the assistance is technological or mechanical, but it may also include other people acting as personal assistants, ASL interpreters, or visual describers. Recently Silvers and Francis (2010, 247) proposed what they call "assistive thinking" through "collaborative trusteeship" for people with cognitive disabilities: "a prosthetic assistive thinking process, enacted through a practice of trust, that reveals and incrementally empowers the personhood of cognitively disabled subjects." Indeed, we might provisionally characterize people with disabilities as those who use prostheses and personal assistance of all kinds.

On that basis, we might imagine a disablist hearing of music that moves beyond the myth of autonomy. Instead of clinging to the assumption that hearing need be a solitary activity, let us imagine that it is something that might be undertaken collaboratively, with assistance either from technology or from another person. Accessibility and accommodation are critical concepts in Disability Studies. The idea is that the social, political, economic, and built environments should be inclusive of people with varying physical and cognitive abilities. Conceptually, the burden thus shifts from the individual (whose impairment is no longer considered a private problem) to the ambient culture (which is now expected to remove barriers to access).

Our theoretical models and our studies of music cognition should be accessible to people with disabilities and to disablist hearing. This may require abandoning the myth of autonomy in the way we think about musical hearing and embracing instead a concept of "universal design," in which differences in hearing are taken account from the very beginning and our theoretical models remain fully accessible to all.[57] That might mean acknowledging hearings that are assisted in one way or another as legitimate forms of music cognition.[58] Autistic listeners might be assisted by a coach or teacher. Deaf listeners might have access to ASL descriptions or, at the very least, to be able to see and feel the music. Blind listeners might have access to Braille notation. And all of these ways of hearing would be considered worthy of inclusion in studies of music cognition. Imagining studies in music cognition as a kind of built environment, and insisting that such an environment follow the precepts of

---

57. According to Morris (2009), the concept of universal design refers to products and environments usable by all people without special adaptation:

> This concept goes beyond the familiar notion of "disabled accessibility," enshrined in the Americans with Disabilities Act. For disabled accessibility, you can have a wheelchair ramp next to a set of stairs. With universal design, you have no stairs to the entrance at all. As a result, everyone can use the same entrance—that's the "universal" in universal design.

58. Readers may recall the discussion in chapter 1 of the reception of the music of Frederick Delius—his collaboration with Eric Fenby in producing his final works led to questions about its authenticity. A criticism rooted in a deeper understanding of disability might understand instead that composition, like hearing, may be a collaborative act.

universal design in being fully accessible to all, would obviously have a radically transformative effect. Even simply contemplating such a possibility makes clear the extent to which the field of music cognition as currently constituted is a highly restrictive enterprise that denies access to people whose style of hearing falls outside of a narrow range.

On second thought, however, it is wrong to suggest that only people with disabilities use prosthetic devices or personal assistance, and wrong to suggest that only disablist hearing is fundamentally collaborative in nature. Indeed, we all use technology to extend our range of activities and to enhance our abilities and we all depend on caregivers—that's the human condition. People with disabilities, however, are generally more aware of this state of interdependency, and the kinds of devices and care they use are specially marked. A better characterization of people with disabilities would be those who use devices and care *beyond the normal*. And disablist hearing can then be defined as hearing that uses devices and personal assistance beyond the normal.

In this context, conventional music notation may be thought of as an assistive, augmentative device. For most listeners, knowledge of music notation enhances their musical abilities, and permits them to make sense of music in ways that are difficult in the absence of notation. In their reliance on traditional notation, normal listeners thus depend on an assistive device, an auditory crutch or prosthesis, in an environment where blind listeners do without. In this sense, music theory itself could be thought of as an assistive or augmentative device, a technology designed to aid and shape hearing. The absence of notation for blind listeners permits the paradoxical observation that, for normal listeners, notation functions as a technological way of gaining access to a built environment, that is, a work of music that would be relatively inaccessible without it. In this view, musical notation (conventional or Braille) should be available to the listeners whose cognition we study.

Disablist hearing would also give listeners better access to other features of musical works, including those (like large-scale key relations and hierarchical structural levels) most valued by theorists. I observed earlier that autistic (absolute pitch) and deaf (visual) listeners would be likely to approach these tasks differently, and with greater success, than normal listeners. The same would be true of listeners with access to notation (conventional or Braille), and even more so for listeners with well-informed personal assistants.

BEYOND NORMAL HEARING

Our standard theoretical models, including especially those grounded in cognitive psychology, not only describe but also enforce normal hearing. Thus, the disablist hearing I am advocating here embodies resistance to the tyranny of the normal. In this respect, I track a central trend throughout Disability Studies (and cultural studies as well). As Carrie Sandahl (2003, 1–2, 26) observes with respect to Disability Studies and Queer Theory:

> Perhaps the most significant similarity between these disciplines, however, is their radical stance toward concepts of normalcy; both argue adamantly against the compulsion to serve norms of all kinds (corporeal, mental, sexual, social, cultural, subcultural, etc.). This stance may even be considered their raison d'être, since both emerged from critiques levied against the normalizing tendencies of their antecedents.... Disability scholars critiqued the fact that disability had long been relegated to academic disciplines (primarily medicine, social sciences, and social services) that considered disabilities "problems" to be cured and the disabled "defectives" to be normalized, not a minority group with its own politics, culture, and history.

In its resistance to the coercive force of normal hearing, my proposed disablist hearing is part of a larger effort within Disability Studies toward empowerment, in which an oppressed and silenced group begins to assert the power of self-representation. Instead of trying to normalize people with disabilities, we listen to what they have to say; instead of turning them into normal hearers, we learn to hear in ways that challenge normal hearing. The goal of the enterprise is not so much about how people with disabilities appear to "us" but how the world looks to people with disabilities. It's about seeing the world from the vantage point of disability. It's about what disability can provide to the listener, not what the listener can do despite disability.

By attending to what I have called disablist hearing, we run the risk of reinforcing the artificial, arbitrary nature of the boundary between normal and disablist hearing, and between normal and disabled bodies. Sacks (2007), perhaps the best-known and widely circulated current discussion of music and disability, operates within the medical model, following a case study approach. He focuses on isolated, deviant individuals, and locates their pathologies within their own bodies. His case studies of freakish hearing actually reinscribe the wall between normal hearing (unexamined, undefined) and abnormal hearing. He is sympathetic to these extraordinary bodies, and his sympathy is a welcome alternative to the pity and scientific objectification that is their usual lot, but he never questions their status as abnormal. My essential point is that the range of human hearing is wider than generally recognized—the boundary between normal and abnormal hearing is a construction, a fiction. We cannot begin to dismantle that wall until we can define better what lies on either side of it.

The social model of disability that I have adopted here leads me to describe disablist hearing as something that emerges within the social grouping of people identified as disabled. From this vantage point, disablist hearing is not a pathology and it does not reside inside the individual body. Rather, it is a mode of cognition and it resides in the relations among people within the group and between groups. Sacks (2007), following the medical model, claims that musical perception is either normal or (because either of excess or deficit) abnormal: "But this wonderful machinery—perhaps because it is so complex and highly developed—is vulnerable to various distortions, excesses, and breakdowns" (xii). My disablist hearings, however, are not distortions, excesses, or breakdowns—they are alternative modes of perception. Like normal hearing, like all hearing, disablist hearing is a cultural artifact, a social construction that emerges among particular social groups, but it is not necessarily exclusively identified with them.

Music theory in general, and music cognition in particular, have usually been essentially conservative enterprises, dedicated to ratifying and rationalizing the status quo. They generally claim that people hear music in only one way, that this is the way they have always heard and always must hear, and that this way of hearing is firmly grounded in nature. False claims of universality are the least attractive feature of the literature on music cognition, which moves too easily from showing that something is widespread to asserting that it is therefore normal, natural, and hardwired into the human brain. In fact, there are many kinds of bodies, many kinds of brains, and many kinds of musical hearing.

In our theorizing, and in our pedagogy, I think we would do well to acknowledge the limitations of normal hearing. The wall of separation between normal and disablist hearing does not benefit those dwelling on either side of it and it has not benefited our larger goal of understanding musical hearing. In dismantling that wall, we have the opportunity to extend our communal sense of how to hear music and to enshrine the full range of human hearings in our theoretical models and in our musical pedagogy.

GLOSSARY OF MUSICAL TERMS

Atonal. Music is *atonal* if it is written without regard to *key*, and if it is impossible for a listener to infer its *key*.

Cadence. A musical punctuation point that conveys a sense of melodic and harmonic arrival.

Chord. A *harmony* of simultaneously sounding tones. In *tonal* music, the principal type of chord is the *major* or *minor triad*.

Chromatic. 1) The five notes not belonging to a given *diatonic* (*major* or *minor*) *scale*; 2) The complete gamut of all twelve tones.

Coda. The optional concluding section of a musical form (literally, "tail"). This section is often used to affirm the principal key (the *tonic*) and to resolve any outstanding structural issues (e.g., "tonal problems").

Consonance. The quality of intervals and chords as relatively harmonious, blended, and stable (compared to *dissonance*).

Counterpoint. The combination of two or more melodic lines. The linear, melodic aspect of music (as opposed to *harmony*, the vertical aspect).

Development. The middle section of a *sonata form*, typically the scene of rapid *modulation* and motivic transformation. More generally, the process of elaborating a musical idea.

Diatonic. The quality of belonging to either a *major* or *minor scale*, without the need for *chromatic* notes. Any *major* or *minor scale* contains seven *diatonic* notes; the remaining five notes are *chromatic*.

Dissonance. The quality of *intervals* and *chords* as relatively inharmonious, unblended, and unstable (compared to *consonance*).

Dominant. Among the notes of a scale, the chords within a key, and the keys within a work, the secondary note, chord, and key in relation to the tonic (the principal note, chord, and key). The dominant is five steps higher than the tonic. In a work in E-flat major, for example, where the tonic note, chord, and key are all E-flat, the dominant note, chord, and key are all B-flat.

Exposition. The first large section of a *sonata form*. Typically, it begins in the *tonic key* and, if the tonic key is *major*, it modulates to the *dominant key*.

Flat. The sign that indicates lowering the *pitch* by the smallest interval (semitone).

Harmony. Notes sounding simultaneously, often grouped together as a *chord*. The vertical aspect of music (as opposed to *counterpoint* and *voice leading*, which represent the horizontal, melodic, linear aspect).

Interval. The distance between two *pitches*, measured in terms of its quality and its size (e.g., "minor third").

Inversion. An operation that transforms a group of tones arranged in register into their mirror image—the *intervals* read from top to bottom are now the *intervals* from bottom to top (and vice versa).

Inversional symmetry. The quality of having the same arrangement of *intervals* reading from top to bottom and bottom to top.

Key. The network of pitch relationships that defines one note and one *harmony* as primary (*tonic*) and assigns subordinate functions to the other notes. There are twelve major and twelve minor keys: C major, C minor, C-sharp major, C-sharp minor, D major, D minor, etc. Music written in a *key* is *tonal* music.

Major. The quality of a *chord* (*harmony*), *scale* or a *key* usually perceived as relatively bright (in contrast to *minor*).

Minor. The quality of a *chord* (*harmony*), *scale* or a *key* usually perceived as relatively dark (in contrast to *major*).

Modulation. The motion from *key* to *key*. All *tonal* works of substantial length involve modulation (changes of key). In a *sonata form*, for example, the first large section (*exposition*) of a piece in a *major key* typically *modulates* from the *tonic* to the *dominant key*.

Notation. A traditional way of writing down music, involving a five-line staff, with notes positioned either on the lines or in the spaces of the staff. Position on the staff indicates *pitch*, with pitches higher (or lower) on the staff corresponding to higher (or lower) register. Traditional notation also conveys information about rhythm.

Pentatonic. A five-note *scale*, equivalent to any transposition of the black keys of the piano keyboard.

Pitch. Any specific point on the continuum from lowest to highest musical sounds. Pitches are normally identified with letter names (A, B, C, D, E, F, G), possibly modified with accidentals (*sharp* signs, which raise the pitch, and *flat* signs, which lower the pitch).

Recapitulation. The concluding section of a *sonata form*. Typically, the recapitulation repeats music from the *exposition*, but instead of *modulating* from *tonic* to *dominant*, as in the exposition, it remains in the tonic *key* throughout. Material heard in the dominant key in the exposition is heard in the tonic key in the recapitulation.

Register. A sector of the range of *pitches* available to a particular instrument or voice, as in a high or low register.

Scale. A repertoire of *pitches* arranged in ascending, stepwise order. The two principal scales of *tonal music* are the *major scale* and the *minor scale*, each with seven notes and a distinctive arrangement of intervals and chords. The *pentatonic scale* is a five-note scale equivalent to any transposition of the black keys of the piano keyboard. The *chromatic scale* consists of all twelve notes.

Series. A precomposed ordering of notes, usually of all twelve notes, for use as the basis of a *twelve-tone* composition.

Sharp. The sign that indicated raising the *pitch* by the smallest *interval* (semitone).

Sonata form. A traditional formal arrangement, the most prevalent and prestigious design of late eighteenth- and early nineteenth-century music. It is usually understood as being in three large sections, an *exposition* (which involves *modulation* from the *tonic key* to a contrasting *key*, usually the *dominant*), a *development* (which involves rapid *modulations* and thematic development), and a *recapitulation* (where the material from the *exposition* that was heard in a *key* other than the *tonic* is now repeated in the *tonic key*). There is an optional, fourth and concluding section, the *coda*.

Tonal. Music is *tonal* if it is written in a particular *key*, or if it moves from key to key. A "tonal problem" is a note that casts doubt on the tonality (sense of key).

Tonic. Among the notes of a *scale*, the *chords* within a *key*, and the keys within a work, the principal note, chord, and key. In a work in E-flat major, for example, the tonic note is E-flat, the tonic chord is the E-flat major chord, and the tonic key is the key of E-flat major.

Triad. A three-note *chord*, *major* or *minor*, which is the basic unit of *harmony* in *tonal music*.

Twelve-tone music. An approach to *atonal* composition devised by Arnold Schoenberg and pursued in a variety of ways by many modernist composers. The melodies and harmonies of a twelve-tone work are derived from a precomposed ordering of the twelve notes of the *chromatic scale*. That ordering is known as a *series*.

Voice leading. The traditional way of connecting *chords* or *harmonies*. If chords or harmonies define the vertical dimension of music, then voice leading defines its horizontal, linear, melodic dimension.

REFERENCES

Adams, Rachel. 2001. *Sideshow U.S.A.: Freaks and the American Cultural Imagination.* Chicago: University of Chicago Press.

Adorno, Theodor. 1988. "Types of Musical Conduct." In *Introduction to the Sociology of Music.* Translated by E. B. Ashton, 1–20. New York: Continuum.

Adorno, Theodor. 1937. "Late Style in Beethoven." In *Essays on Music,* ed. Richard Leppert. Trans. Susan H. Gillespie, 564–68. Berkeley and Los Angeles: University of California Press, 2002.

Alajouanine, Théophile. 1948. "Aphasia and Artistic Realization." *Brain* 71: 229–41.

Aldwell, Edward and Carl Schachter. 1989. *Harmony and Voice Leading,* 2d ed. New York: Harcourt Brace Jovanovich.

Almen, Byron. 2008. *A Theory of Musical Narrative.* Bloomington: Indiana University Press.

Alvin, Juliette and Auriel Warwick. 1991. *Music Therapy for the Autistic Child,* 2d ed. Oxford: Oxford University Press.

Antokoletz, Elliott. 1984. *The Music of Bartók: A Study of Tonality and Progression in Twentieth-Century Music.* Berkeley and Los Angeles: University of California Press.

Archibald, Bruce. 1972. "Some Thoughts on Symmetry in Early Webern, Op. 5, No. 2." *Perspectives of New Music* 10(2): 159–63.

Ashby, Arved. 2004. "Intention and Meaning in Modernist Music." In *The Pleasure of Modernist Music: Listening, Meaning, Intention, Ideology,* ed. Arved Ashby, 23–45. Rochester, N.Y.: University of Rochester Press.

Auner, Joseph, ed. 2003. *A Schoenberg Reader: Documents of a Life.* New Haven, Conn.: Yale University Press.

Aviv, Rachel. 2010. "Listening to Braille." *Sunday New York Times Magazine,* January 3, 2010: 42–45.

Ayotte, Julie et al. 2002. "Congenital Amusia: A Group Study of Adults Afflicted with a Music-Specific Disorder." *Brain* 125(2): 238–51.

Ayrton, William. 1823. *The Harmonicon: A Journal of Music.* London: William Pinnock.

Bahan, Benjamin. 2006. "Face-to-Face Tradition in the American Deaf Community Dynamics of the Teller, the Tale, and the Audience." In *Signing the Body Poetic: Essays on American Sign Language Literature,* ed. H-Dirksen L. Bauman, Jennifer L. Nelson, and Heidi M. Rose, 21–50. Berkeley and Los Angeles: University of California Press.

Bahan, Benjamin. 2008. "Upon the Formation of a Visual Variety of the Human Race." In *Open Your Eyes: Deaf Studies Talking,* ed. H-Dirksen L. Bauman, 83–99. Minneapolis: University of Minnesota Press.

Bailey, Kathryn. 1991. *The Twelve-Note Music of Anton Webern.* Cambridge: Cambridge University Press.

Bailey, Walter. 1984. *Programmatic Elements in the Works of Schoenberg.* Ann Arbor, MI: UMI Research Press.

Barasch, Moshe. 2001. *Blindness: The History of a Mental Image in Western Thought*. New York: Routledge.

Baron-Cohen, Simon, ed. 1993. *Understanding Other Minds: Perspectives from Autism*. Oxford: Oxford University Press.

Baron-Cohen, Simon. 1997. *Mindblindness: An Essay on Autism and Theory of Mind*. Cambridge, Mass.: MIT Press.

Baron-Cohen, Simon. 2001. "Theory of Mind and Autism: a Review." Special Issue of *International Review of Mental Retardation* 23: 169–84.

Baron-Cohen, Simon. 2004. *The Essential Difference*. London: Penguin.

Bauer, Amy. 2004. "'Tone-Color, Movement, Changing Harmonic Planes': Cognition, Constraints, and Conceptual Blends in Modernist Music." In *The Pleasure of Modernist Music: Listening, Meaning, Intention, Ideology*, ed. Arved Ashby, 121–52. Rochester, N.Y.: University of Rochester Press.

Bauman, H-Dirksen L. 2008. "Introduction: Listening to Deaf Studies." In *Open Your Eyes: Deaf Studies Talking*, ed. H-Dirksen L. Bauman, 1–34. Minneapolis: University of Minnesota Press.

Baynton, Douglas. 2001. "Disability and the Justification of Inequality in American History." In *The New Disability History: American Perspectives*, ed. Paul Longmore and Lauri Umansky, 33–57. New York: New York University Press.

Baynton, Douglas. 2008. "Beyond Culture: Deaf Studies and the Deaf Body." In *Open Your Eyes: Deaf Studies Talking*, ed. H-Dirksen L. Bauman, 293–313. Minneapolis: University of Minnesota Press.

Bazzana, Kevin. 1997. *Glenn Gould, The Performer in the Work: A Study in Performance Practice*. Oxford: Clarendon Press.

Bazzana, Kevin. 2004. *Wondrous Strange: The Life and Art of Glenn Gould*. Oxford: Oxford University Press.

Beecham, Thomas. 1959. *Frederick Delius*. London: Hutchinson.

Belmonte, Matthew K. 2008. "Human, but More So: What the Autistic Brain Tells Us about the Process of Narrative." In *Autism and Representation*, ed. Mark Osteen, 166–80. New York: Routledge.

Bernstein, David. 1993. "Symmetry and Symmetrical Inversion in Turn-of-the-Century Theory and Practice." In *Music Theory and the Exploration of the Past*, ed. Christopher Hatch and David Bernstein, 377–408. Chicago: University of Chicago Press.

Bevan, Peter Gilroy. 1998. "Adversity: Schubert's illnesses and their background." In *Schubert Studies*, ed. Brian Newbould, 244–66. Aldershot, England: Ashgate.

Bharucha, Jamshed and Carol Krumhansl. 1983. "The representation of harmonic structure in music: Hierarchies of stability as a function of context." *Cognition* 13(1): 63–102.

Bigand, Emmanuel and Bénédicte Poulin-Charronnat. 2009. "Tonal Cognition." In *The Oxford Handbook of Music Psychology*, ed. Susan Hallam, Ian Cross, and Michael Thaut, 59–71. Oxford: Oxford University Press.

Bloom, Harold. 1973. *The Anxiety of Influence: A Theory of Poetry*. Oxford: Oxford University Press.

Bloom, Harold. 1975. *A Map of Misreading*. Oxford: Oxford University Press.

Bloom, Harold. 1976. *Poetry and Repression: Revisionism from Blake to Stevens*. New Haven, Conn.: Yale University Press.

Bloom, Harold. 1983. *Kaballah and Criticism*. New York: Continuum.

Blume, Friedrich. 1979. *Classic and Romantic Music: A Comprehensive Survey*, translated by M. D. Herter Norton. London: Faber & Faber.

Bogdan, Robert. 1988. *Freak Show: Presenting Human Oddities for Amusement and Profit*. Chicago: University of Chicago Press.

Bonds, Mark Evan. 1991. *Wordless Rhetoric: Musical Form and the Metaphor of the Oration.* Cambridge, Mass.: Harvard University Press.

Bónis, Ferenc. 1963. "Quotations in Bartók's Music." *Studia Musicologica* 5: 355–82.

Boros, James. 1995. "A 'New Totality'?" *Perspectives of New Music* 33(1–2): 538–53.

Boyer, John. 1995. *Culture and Political Crisis in Viena: Christian Socialism in Power, 1897–1918.* Chicago: University of Chicago Press.

Braddock, David and Susan Parish. 2001. "An Institutional History of Disability." In *Handbook of Disability Studies*, ed. Gary Albrecht, Katherine Seelman, and Michael Bury, 11–68. Thousand Oaks, Calif.: Sage.

Brandenburg, Sieghard. 1982. "The Historical Background to the 'Heiliger Dankgesang' in Beethoven's A-Minor Quartet, Op. 132." In *Beethoven Studies*, vol. 3, ed. Alan Tyson, 161–92. Cambridge: Cambridge University Press.

Branson, Jan and Don Miller. 2002. *Damned for Their Difference: The Cultural Construction of Deaf People as Disabled.* Washington, D.C.: Gallaudet University Press.

Brendel, Alfred. 1990. *Music Sounded Out.* London: Robson Books.

Brookes, Martin. 2004. *Extreme Measures: The Dark Visions and Bright Ideas of Francis Galton.* New York: Bloomsbury.

Brower, Candace. 1997–98. "Pathway, Blockage, and Containment in Density 21.5." *Theory and Practice* 22–23: 35–54.

Brower, Candace. 2000. "A Cognitive Theory of Musical Meaning." *Journal of Music Theory* 44(2): 323–80.

Brower, Candace. 2008. "Paradoxes of Pitch Space," *Music Analysis* 27(1): 51–106.

Brown, Walter A. et al. 2003. "Autism-Related Language, Personality, and Cognition in People with Absolute Pitch: Results of a Preliminary Study." *Journal of Autism and Developmental Disorders* 33(2): 163–67.

Burnham, Scott. 1995. *Beethoven Hero.* Princeton, N.J.: Princeton University Press.

Burnham, Scott. 2001a. "Beethoven, Ludwig van: Posthumous Influence and Reception." In *The New Grove Dictionary of Music and Musicians*, 2d ed., ed. Stanley Sadie, vol. 3, 110–14. London: Macmillan.

Burnham, Scott. 2001b. "The Second Nature of Sonata Form." In *Music Theory and Natural Order from the Renaissance to the Early Twentieth Century*, ed. Suzannah Clark and Alexander Rehding, 111–41. Cambridge: Cambridge University Press.

Burnham, Scott. 2002. "Form." In *The Cambridge History of Music Theory*, ed. Thomas Christensen, 880–906. Cambridge: Cambridge University Press.

Burnham, Scott. 2006. "Late Styles." Paper presented at "'New Paths': Robert Schumann, 1848–1856," McGill University, Toronto, Canada.

Burstein, L. Poundie. 2006. "*Les chansons des fous*: On the Edge of Madness with Alkan." In *Sounding Off: Theorizing Disability in Music*, ed. Neil Lerner and Joseph N. Straus, 187–98. New York: Routledge.

Busse-Berger, Anna Maria. 2005. *Medieval Music and the Art of Memory.* Berkeley and Los Angeles: University of California Press.

Butler, David. 1992. *The Musician's Guide to Perception and Cognition.* New York: Schirmer Books.

Butler, Judith. 1993. *Bodies that Matter: On the Discursive Limits of "Sex".* New York: Routledge.

Butler, Judith. 1999. *Gender Trouble: Feminism and the Subversion of Identity.* New York: Routledge.

Cameron, Lindsley. 1998. *The Music of Light: the Extraordinary Story of Hikari and Kenzaburo Oe.* New York: Free Press.

Canguilhem, Georges. 1991. *On the Normal and the Pathological*, trans. R. Fawcett. New York: Zone Books.

Caplin, William. 1998. *Classical Form: A Theory of Formal Functions for the Instrumental Music of Haydn, Mozart, and Beethoven.* Oxford: Oxford University Press.

Carpenter, Patricia. 1988. "A Problem in Organic Form: Schoenberg's Tonal Body." *Theory and Practice* 13: 31–64.

Carruthers, Mary. 1992. *The Book of Memory: A Study of Memory in Medieval Culture.* Cambridge: Cambridge University Press.

Cherlin, Michael. 1991. "Dramaturgy and Mirror Imagery in Schoenberg's Moses und Aron: Two Paradigmatic Interval Palindromes." *Perspectives of New Music* 29(2): 50–71.

Cherlin, Michael. 1998. "Memory and Rhetorical Trope in Schoenberg's String Trio." *Journal of the American Musicological Society* 51: 559–602.

Cherlin, Michael. 2007. *Schoenberg's Musical Imagination.* Cambridge: Cambridge University Press.

Chew, Kristina. 2008. "Fractioned Idiom: Metonymy and the Language of Autism." In *Autism and Representation*, ed. Mark Osteen, 133–44. New York: Routledge.

Cohen, David. 1993. "Metaphysics, Ideology, Discipline: Consonance, Dissonance, and the Foundations of Western Polyphony." *Theoria* 7: 1–85.

Cohen, Deborah. 2001. *The War Come Home: Disabled Veterans in Britain and Germany, 1914–1939.* Berkeley and Los Angeles: University of California Press.

Cohn, Richard. 1999. "As Wonderful as Star Clusters: Instruments for Gazing at Tonality in Schubert." *Nineteenth-Century Music* 22: 213–32.

Cone, Edward. 1982. "Schubert's Promissory Note: An Exercise in Musical Hermeneutics." *Nineteenth-Century Music* 5(3): 233–41.

Connelly, Frances, ed. 2003. *Modern Art and the Grotesque.* Cambridge: Cambridge University Press.

Cook, Nicholas. 1987. "The perception of large-scale tonal closure." *Music Perception* 5(2): 197–205.

Cook, Nicholas. 1994. "Perception: A Perspective from Music Theory." In *Musical Perceptions*, ed. Rita Aiello, 64–98. New York: Oxford University Press.

Copland, Aaron and Vivian Perlis. 1989. *Copland Since 1943.* New York: St. Martin's Press.

Corker, Mairian and Sally French. 1999. "Reclaiming Discourse in Disability Studies." In *Disability Discourse*, ed. Mairian Corker and Sally French, 1–12. Buckingham, England: Open University Press.

Couser, Thomas G. 1997. *Recovering Bodies: Illness, Disability and Life Writing.* Madison: University of Wisconsin Press.

Craft, Robert. 1994. *Stravinsky: Chronicle of a Friendship 1948–1971.* New York: Knopf, 1972; rev. and expanded ed.. Nashville, Tenn.: Vanderbilt University Press.

Crist, Elizabeth and Wayne Shirley, eds. 2006. *The Selected Correspondence of Aaron Copland.* New Haven, Conn.: Yale University Press.

Cusick, Suzanne. 1994. "On a Lesbian Relationship with Music: A Serious Effort Not to Think Straight." In *Queering the Pitch: The New Gay and Lesbian Musicology*, ed. Philip Brett, Elizabeth Wood, and Gary Thomas, 67–84. New York: Routledge.

Daverio, John. 1997. *Robert Schumann: Herald of a "New Poetic Age."* New York: Oxford University Press.

Davidson, Michael. 2008. *Concerto for the Left Hand: Disability and the Defamiliar Body.* Ann Arbor: University of Michigan Press.

Davies, Peter. 2001. *Beethoven in Person: His Deafness, Illnesses, and Death.* Westport, Conn.: Greenwood Press.

Davies, Benjamin K. 2007. "The Structuring of Tonal Space in Webern's Six Bagatelles for String Quartet, Op. 9." *Music Analysis* 26(1–2) (2007): 25–58.

Davis, Lennard. 1995. *Enforcing Normalcy: Disability, Deafness, and the Body.* London: Verso.

Davis, Lennard. 1997a. "Constructing Normalcy: The Bell Curve, the Novel, and the Invention of the Disabled Body in the Nineteenth Century." In *The Disability Studies Reader*, ed. Lennard Davis, 9–28. New York: Routledge.

Davis, Lennard. 1997b. "Nude Venuses, Medusa's Body, and Phantom Limbs: Disability and Visuality." In *The Body and Physical Difference*, ed. David Mitchell and Sharon Snyder, 51–70. Ann Arbor: University of Michigan Press.

Davis, Lennard. 2002. *Bending Over Backwards: Disability, Dismodernism and Other Difficult Positions*. New York: New York University Press.

Davis, Lennard. 2003. "Identity Politics, Disability, and Culture." In *Handbook of Disability Studies*, ed. Gary Albrecht, Katherine Seelman, and Michael Bury, 535–45. Thousand Oaks, Calif.: Sage.

Davis, Lennard. 2008. *Obsession: A History*. Chicago: University of Chicago Press.

Davis, John and M. Grace Baron. 2006. "Blind Tom: A Celebrated Slave Pianist Coping with the Stress of Autism." In *Stress and Coping in Autism*, ed. M. Grace Baron et al., 96–126. New York: Oxford University Press.

DeBellis, Mark. 2002. "Musical Analysis as Articulation." *Journal of Aesthetics and Art Criticism* 60(2):119–35.

Deliège, Irene. 1987. "Grouping Conditions in Listening to Music: An Approach to Lerdahl and Jackendoff's Grouping Preference Rules." *Music Perception* 4: 325–59.

Deutsch, Diana. 1999. "The Processing of Pitch Combinations." In *The Psychology of Music*, 2d ed., ed. Diana Deutsch, 349–411. San Diego, Calif.: Academic Press.

Deutsch, Helen. 2002. "Exemplary Aberration: Samuel Johnson and the English Canon." In *Disability Studies: Enabling the Humanities*, ed. Sharon L. Snyder, Brenda Jo Brueggemann, and Rosemarie Garland-Thomson, 197–210. New York: Modern Language Association of America.

Dolmage, Jay. 2005. "Between the Valley and the Field: Metaphor and Disability." *Prose Studies* 27(1–2): 108–19.

Downs, Philip G. 1970. "Beethoven's 'New Way' and the Eroica." *Musical Quarterly* 56: 585–604.

Draughon, Francesca. 2003. "Dance of Decadence: Class, Gender, and Modernity in the Scherzo of Mahler's Ninth Symphony." *Journal of Musicology* 20(3): 388–413.

Dregni, Michael. 2004. *Django: The Life and Music of a Gypsy Legend*. New York: Oxford University Press.

Dubiel, Joseph. 1999. "Composer, Theorist, Composer/Theorist." In *Rethinking Music*, ed. Nicholas Cook and Mark Everist, 262–86. New York: Oxford University Press.

Dubiel, Joseph. 2008. "A Modification to Consider in Layer Theories of Tonality." Unpublished ms.

Ealy, George. 1994. "Of Ear Trumpets and a Resonance Plate: Early Aids and Beethoven's Hearing Perception." *Nineteenth-Century Music* 17(3): 262–73.

Earp, Lawrence. 1993. "Tovey's 'Cloud' in the First Movement of the *Eroica*: An Analysis Based on Sketches for the Development and Coda." In *Beethoven Forum*, vol. 2, ed. Christopher Reynolds, Lewis Lockwood, and James Webster, 66–76. Lincoln: University of Nebraska Press.

Ebenstein, William. 2006. "Toward an Archetypal Psychology of Disability Based on the Hephaestus Myth." *Disability Studies Quarterly* 26(4).

Eitan, Zohar and Roni Granot. 2006. "How Music Moves: Musical Parameters and Listeners' Images of Motion." *Music Perception* 23(3): 221–47.

Eitan, Zohar and Renee Timmers. 2010. "Beethoven's Last Piano Sonata and Those Who Follow Crocodiles: Cross-Domain Mappings of Auditory Pitch in a Musical Context." *Cognition* 114/3: 405–422.

Ellinwood, Leonard. 1936. "Francesco Landini and His Music." *Musical Quarterly* 22(2): 190–216.

Epstein, David. 1987. *Beyond Orpheus: Studies in Musical Structure*. Cambridge, Mass.: MIT Press.

Feldmann, H. 1971. "The Otological Aspects of Bedrich Smetana's Disease," trans. Ernst Levin. *Music Review* 32(3): 233–47.

Fenby, Eric. 1981. *Delius as I Knew Him* (1936). Cambridge: Cambridge University Press.

Ferris, Jim. 2005. "Aesthetic Distance and the Fiction of Disability." In *Commotion: Disability and Performance*, eds. Carrie Sandahl and Philip Auslander, 56–68. Ann Arbor: University of Michigan Press.

Fineman, Martha Albertson. 2004. *The Autonomy Myth: A Theory of Dependency*. New York: New Press.

Fisher, George and Judy Lochhead. 2002. "Analyzing from the Body." *Theory and Practice* 27: 37–67.

Fisk, Charles. 2001. *Returning Cycles: Contexts for the Interpretation of Schubert's Impromptus and Last Sonatas*. Berkeley and Los Angeles: University of California Press.

Fitzgerald, Michael 2004. *Autism and Creativity: Is there a Link between Autism in Men and Exceptional Creativity?* New York: Routledge.

Floros, Constantin. 1978. *Beethovens Eroica und Prometheus Musik*. Wilhelmshaven, Germany: Heinrichshofen Verlag.

Foucault, Michel. 1978. *The History of Sexuality: An Introduction*. Reprint, New York: Random House, 1990.

Frank, Arthur W. 1995. *The Wounded Storyteller: Body, Illness, and Ethics*. Chicago: University of Chicago Press.

Frith, Uta. 2003. *Autism: Explaining the Enigma*, 2d ed. Oxford: Blackwell.

Frith, Uta and Francesca Happé. 1999. "Theory of Mind and Self-Consciousness: What is It Like to Be Autistic?" *Mind and Language* 14(1): 1–22.

Fullerton, Graeme. 2005. *The Grotesque in 20th-Century Opera*. Ph.D. diss., City University of New York.

Gaab Nadine et al. 2006. "Neural Correlates of Absolute Pitch Differ between Blind and Sighted Musicians." *Neuroreport* 17:1853–57.

Garland-Thomson, Rosemarie, ed. 1996. *Freakery: Cultural Spectacles of the Extraordinary Body*. New York: New York University Press.

Garland-Thomson, Rosemarie. 1997a. *Extraordinary Bodies: Figuring Physical Disability in American Culture and Literature*. New York: Columbia University Press.

Garland-Thomson, Rosemarie. 1997b. "Feminist Theory, the Body, and the Disabled Figure." In *The Disability Studies Reader*, ed. Lennard Davis, 279–94. New York: Routledge.

Garland-Thomson, Rosemarie. 2001. "Seeing the Disabled: Visual Rhetorics of Disability in Popular Photography." In *The New Disability History: American Perspectives*, ed. Paul K. Longmore and Lauri Umansky, 335–74. New York: New York University Press.

Garland-Thomson, Rosemarie. 2004a. "The Cultural Logic of Euthanasia: 'Sad Fancyings' in Herman Melville's 'Bartelby.'" *American Literature* 76(4): 777–806.

Garland-Thomson, Rosemarie. 2004b. "Integrating Disability, Transforming Feminist Theory." In *Gendering Disability*, ed. Bonnie G. Smith and Beth Hutchison, 73–106. New Brunswick, N.J.: Rutgers University Press.

Garland-Thomson, Rosemarie. 2005. "Dares to Stare: Disabled Women Performance Artists and the Dynamics of Staring." In *Bodies in Commotion: Disability and Performance*, ed. Carrie Sandahl and Philip Auslander, 30–41. Ann Arbor: University of Michigan Press.

Garland-Thomson, Rosemarie. 2009. *Staring: How We Look*. New York: Oxford University Press.

Gerber, David, ed. 2000. *Disabled Veterans in History*. Ann Arbor: University of Michigan Press.

Gereben, Janos. 2002. "Quasthoff: A Hero's Journey Transforms the Festival Concert Hall." *Oakland Post*, July 7, 2002.

Gerland, Gunilla. 1997. *A Real Person: Life On the Outside*, trans. Joan Tate. London: Souvenir Press.

Gibbs, Christopher. 2000. *The Life of Schubert*. Cambridge: Cambridge University Press.

Gibbs, Raymond. 1994. *The Poetics of Mind: Figurative Thought, Language, and Understanding*. Cambridge: Cambridge University Press.

Gillies, Malcom. 2001. "Bartók in America. " In *The Cambridge Companion to Bartók*, ed. Amanda Bayley, 190–201. Cambridge: Cambridge University Press.

Gimbel, Allen. 2010. "Allan Pettersson as a Topic for Disability Studies." Unpublished paper.

Gleick, Elizabeth. 1997. "Triumph of the Spirit: German Singer Thomas Quasthoff is Thrilling Audiences with his Voice—and his Courage." *Time Magazine* 149(26), June 30, 1997.

Glennie, Evelyn. 1990. *Good Vibrations: An Autobiography*. London: Arrow Books.

Glennie, Evelyn. 2010a. "Hearing Essay." Retrieved October 1, 2009 from http://www.evelyn.co.uk/Evelyn_old/live/hearing_essay.htm.

Glennie, Evelyn. 2010b. "Disability Essay." Retrieved October 1, 2009 from http://www.evelyn.co.uk/Evelyn_old/live/disability_essay.htm.

Goffman, Erving. 1963. *Stigma: Notes on the Management of Spoiled Identity*. New York: Simon & Schuster.

Goldmark, Daniel. 2006. "Stuttering in American Popular Song, 1890–1930." In *Sounding Off: Theorizing Disability in Music*, ed. Neil Lerner and Joseph N. Straus, 75–90. New York: Routledge.

Grainger, Percy. 1976. "The Personality of Frederick Delius." In *A Delius Companion*, ed. Christopher Redwood, 117–30. London: John Calder.

Grandin, Temple. 1995. *Thinking in Pictures, and Other Reports from my Life with Autism*. New York: Doubleday.

Grave, Floyd. 2008. "Recuperation, Transformation, and the Transcendence of Major over Minor in the Finale of Haydn's String Quartet, Op. 76, No. 1." *Eighteenth-Century Music* 5(1): 27–50.

Gray, Cecil. 1976. "Memories of Delius. " In *A Delius Companion*, ed. Christopher Redwood, 135–45. London: John Calder.

Grigely, Joseph. 2000. "Postcards to Sophie Calle." In *Points of Contact: Disability, Art, and Culture*, ed. Susan Crutchfield and Marcy Epstein, 31–58. Ann Arbor: University of Michigan Press.

Grinker, Roy. 2007. *Unstrange Minds: Remapping the World of Autism*. New York: Basic Books.

Grosz, Elizabeth. 1994. *Volatile Bodies: Towards a Corporeal Feminism*. Bloomington: Indiana University Press.

Grove, Thelma. 1987. "Barnaby Rudge: A Case Study in Autism." *Dickensian* 83: 139–48.

Gur, Golan. 2008. "Body, Forces, and Paths." *Music Theory Online* 14(1).

Hacking, Ian. 1998. *Mad Travelers: Reflections on the Reality of Transient Mental Illnesses*. Cambridge, Mass.: Harvard University Press.

Haimo, Ethan. 1998. "The Late Twelve-Tone Compositions." In *The Arnold Schoenberg Companion*, ed. Walter Bailey, 157–76. Westport, Conn.: Greenwood Press.

Hamilton, Roy, Alvaro Pascual-Leone, and Gottfried Schlaug. 2004. "Absolute Pitch in Blind Musicians." *Neuroreport* 15(5): 803–806.

Happé, Francesca. 2005. "The Weak Central Coherence Account of Autism." In *Handbook of Autism and Pervasive Developmental Disorders*, 3d ed., ed. Fred R. Volkmar, Rhea Paul, Ami Klin, and Donald Cohen, 640–49. Hoboken, N.J.: Wiley.

Hatten, Robert. 2004. *Interpreting Musical Gestures, Topics, and Tropes: Mozart, Beethoven, Schubert.* Bloomington: Indiana University Press.

Hawkins, Anne Hunsaker. 1999. *Reconstructing Illness: Studies in Pathography,* 2d ed. West Lafayette, Ind.: Purdue University Press.

Hayden, Deborah. 2003. *Pox: Genius, Madness, and the Mysteries of Syphilis.* New York: Basic Books.

Headlam, Dave. 2006. "Learning to Hear Autistically." In *Sounding Off: Theorizing Disability in Music,* ed. Neil Lerner and Joseph N. Straus, 109–20. New York: Routledge.

Healy, Maureen. 2004. *Vienna and the Fall of the Hapsburg Empire: Total War and Everyday Life in World War I.* Cambridge: Cambridge University Press.

Henahan, Donal. 1970. "When Toby Says it was Terrific, Then I'm Happy." *New York Times,* March 8, 1970: D15, 24.

Hepokoski, James. 2001–2002. "Back and Forth from Egmont: Beethoven, Mozart, and the Nonresolving Recapitulation." *Nineteenth-Century Music* 25(2–3): 127–54.

Hepokoski, James. 2002. "Beyond the Sonata Principle." *Journal of the American Musicological Society* 55(1): 91–154.

Hepokoski, James and Warren Darcy. 1997. "The Medial Caesura and Its Role in the Eighteenth-Century Sonata Exposition." *Music Theory Spectrum* 19: 115–54.

Hepokoski, James and Warren Darcy. 2006. *Elements of Sonata Theory: Norms, Types, and Deformations in the Late-Eighteenth Century Sonata.* New York: Oxford University Press.

Hermelin, Beate et al. 1987. "Musical Inventiveness of Five Idiots-Savants." *Psychological Medicine* 17: 79–90.

Hockenberry, John. 1995. *Moving Violations (A Memoir): War Zones, Wheelchairs, and Declations of Independence.* New York: Hyperion.

Honisch, Stefan Sunandan. 2009. "Re-narrating Disability" through Musical Performance." *Music Theory Online* 15(3–4).

Honisch, Stefan Sunandan. 2010. "Claiming the Speechless Space Surrounding Us: Tempo, Rhythm and Phrasing as Metaphors of Embodied Experience." Paper presented at the City University of New York Symposium on Music and Disability, January 2010.

Hook, Julian. 2002. "Hearing with our Eyes: The Geometry of Tonal Space." In *Bridges: Mathematical Connections in Art, Music, and Science* 5: 123–34.

Horden, Peregrine, ed. 2000. *Music as Medicine: the History of Music Therapy since Antiquity.* Aldershot, England: Ashgate.

Howe, Blake. 2010a. *Problematic Embodiments: Locating Disability, Disease, and Disfigurement in Music.* Ph.D. diss., City University of New York, New York.

Howe, Blake. 2010b. "Paul Wittgenstein and the Performance Of Disability." *Journal of Musicology* 27/2: 135–80.

Hughes, Allen. 1968. "Maazel Conducts at Carnegie Hall," *New York Times,* January 31, 1968: 26.

Hughes, Allen. 1969. "Perlman is Last in Hunter Series." *New York Times,* April 28, 1969: 34.

Hughes, Timothy. 2003. *Groove and Flow: Six Analytical Essays on the Music of Stevie Wonder.* Ph.D. diss., University of Washington, Seattle, Wash.

Hurt-Thaut, Corene. 2009. "Clinical Practice in Music Therapy." In *The Oxford Handbook of Music Psychology,* ed. Susan Hallam, Ian Cross, and Michael Thaut, 503–14. Oxford: Oxford University Press.

Hyer, Brian. 1995. "Second Immediacies in the 'Eroica.'" In *Music Theory in the Age of Romanticism,* ed. Ian Bent, 77–104. Cambridge: Cambridge University Press.

Jakobson, Roman. 1971. "Two Aspects of Language and Two Types Of Aphasic Disturbances." *Fundamentals of Language,* 55–82. The Hague, The Netherlands: Mouton.

James, Michael. 2001. "Reinhardt, Django." In *The New Grove Dictionary of Music and Musicians,* 2d ed. London: Macmillan.

Jamison, Kay Redfield. 1996. *Touched with Fire: Manic-Depressive Illness and the Artistic Temperament*. New York: Free Press.

Jander, Owen. 2000. " 'Let Your Deafness No Longer Be a Secret—Even in Art': Self-Portraiture and the Third Movement of the C-Minor Symphony." In *Beethoven Forum 8*, ed. Lewis Lockwood, Christopher Reynolds, and Elaine R. Sisman, 25–70. Lincoln: University of Nebraska Press.

Jefferson, Alan. 1972. *Delius*. London: Dent.

Jensen, Eric Frederick. 2001. *Schumann*. Oxford: Oxford University Press.

Jensen-Moulton, Stephanie. 2006. "Finding Autism in the Composition of a 19th-Century Prodigy." In *Sounding Off: Theorizing Disability in Music*, ed. Neil Lerner and Joseph N. Straus, 199–216. New York: Routledge.

Jers, Norbert. 1976. *Igor Strawinskys Späte Zwölftonwerke (1958–1966)*. Regensburg: Gustav Bosse Verlag.

Johnson, Harriet McBryde. 2005. *Too Late to Die Young: Nearly True Tales from a Life*. New York: Henry Holt.

Johnson, Mark. 1987. *The Body in the Mind: The Bodily Basis of Meaning, Imagination, and Reason*. Chicago: University of Chicago Press.

Johnson, Mark. 1997–98. "Embodied Musical Meaning." *Theory and Practice* 22–23: 95–102.

Johnson, Shersten. 2008. "Disintermediation of Music Spaces: Re(con)figuring Visual, Aural, and Tactile Interactions." Paper presented to the Society for Disability Studies, New York.

Johnson, Shersten. 2009. "Notational Systems and Conceptualizing Music: A Case Study of Print and Braille Notation. *Music Theory Online* 15(3).

Jourdan-Morhange, Hélène. 1945. *Ravel et Nous*. Geneva, Switzerland: Éditions du Milieu du Monde.

Kamien, Roger. 2000. "Phrase, period, theme." In *The Cambridge Companion to Beethoven*, ed. Glenn Stanley, 64–83. Cambridge: Cambridge University Press.

Kanner, Leo. 1943. "Autistic Disturbances of Affective Contact." *Nervous Child* 2: 217–50.

Kanner, Leo. 1949. "Problems of Nosology and Psychodynamics of Early Infantile Autism." *American Journal of Orthopsychiatry* 19: 425.

Katz, Derek. 1997. "Smetana's Second String Quartet: Voice of Madness or Triumph of Spirit?" *Musical Quarterly* 81(4): 516–36.

Keller, Hans. 1994. "Principles of Composition (1960)." In *Essays on Music*, ed. Irene Samuel, Bayan Northcott, and Christopher Wintle, 212–32. Cambridge: Cambridge University Press.

Kellow, Brian. 2005. "The Key to Tobias." *Opera News* 70(2): 16–22.

Kerman, Joseph. 1979. *The Beethoven Quartets*. New York: Norton.

Kerman, Joseph. 1986. "A Romantic Detail in Schubert's 'Schwanengesang.'" In *Schubert: Critical and Analytical Studies*, ed. Walter Frisch, 48–64. Lincoln: University of Nebraska Press.

Kinderman, William. 1997. "Wandering Archetypes in Schubert's Instrumental Music." *Nineteenth-Century Music* 21(2): 208–22.

Kinderman, William. 2009. *Beethoven*, 2d ed. Oxford: Oxford University Press.

Kleege, Georgina. 1999. *Sight Unseen*. New Haven, Conn.: Yale University Press.

Klumpenhouwer, Henry. 2005. "Review of Lerdahl, *Tonal Pitch Space*." *Journal of the American Musicological Society* 58(2): 488–96.

Knittel, K. M. 1995. "Imitation, Individuality, and Illness: Behind Beethoven's Three Styles." *Beethoven Forum* 4: 17–36.

Knittell, K. M. 1998. "Wagner, Deafness, and the Reception of Beethoven's Late Style." *Journal of American Musicological Society* 51(1): 49–82.

Knittel, K. M. 2002. "The Construction of Beethoven." In *The Cambridge History of Nineteenth-Century Music*, ed. Jim Samson, 118–56. Cambridge: Cambridge University Press.

Kopp, David. 2002. *Chromatic Transformations in Nineteenth-Century Music*. Cambridge: Cambridge University Press.

Korsyn, Kevin. 1991. "Towards a New Poetics of Musical Influence." *Music Analysis* 10(1–2): 3–72.

Kriegel, Leonard. 1987. "The Cripple in Literature." In *Images of Disability, Disabling Images*, ed. A. Gartner & T. Joe, 31–46. New York: Praeger.

Kriegsman, Alan. 1971. "Perlman: No Bow to a Handicap." *Washington Post*, January 13, 1971: B1.

Krumhansl, Carol. 1990. *Cognitive Foundations of Musical Pitch*. Oxford: Oxford University Press.

Kuppers, Petra. 2001. *Disability and Contemporary Performance: Bodies on Edge*. London: Routledge.

Kutchins, Herb and Stuart A. Kirk. 1997. *Making us Crazy: DSM: The Psychiatric Bible and the Creation of Mental Disorders*. New York: Free Press.

Kuusisto, Stephen. 2006. *Eavesdropping: A Memoir of Blindness and Listening*. New York: Norton.

LaCom, Cindy. 1997. "'It is More than Lame': Female Disability, Sexuality, and the Maternal in the Nineteenth-Century Novel." In *The Body and Physical Difference: Discourses of Disability*, ed. David Mitchell and Sharon Snyder, 189–201. Ann Arbor: University of Michigan Press.

Lakoff, George. 1987. *Women, Fire, and Dangerous Things: What Categories Reveal about the Mind*. Chicago: University of Chicago Press.

Lakoff, George and Mark Johnson. 1980. *Metaphors We Live By*. Chicago: University of Chicago Press.

Lane, Harlan. 1984. *When the Mind Hears: A History of the Deaf*. New York: Random House.

Large, Brian. 1970. *Smetana*. New York: Praeger.

Larkin, Edward. 1970. "Beethoven's Medical History." In Martin Cooper, *Beeethoven: The Last Decade, 1817–1827*, 439–66. New York: Oxford University Press.

Larkin, Kathy. 1986. "A Virtuoso at Clearing Barriers." *Chicago Tribune*, July 3, 1986: N3.

Le Guin, Elizabeth. 2002. "'One Says That One Weeps, but One Does Not Weep': Sensible, Grotesque, and Mechanical Embodiments in Boccherini's Chamber Music." *Journal of the American Musicological Society* 55(2): 207–54.

LeGuin, Elisabeth. 2004. "One Bar in Eight: Debussy and the Death of Description." In *Beyond Structural Listening?: Postmodern Modes of Hearing*, ed. Andrew Dell'Antonio, 233–51. Berkeley and Los Angeles: University of California Press.

LeGuin, Elisabeth. 2006. *Boccherini's Body: An Essay in Carnal Musicology*. Berkeley and Los Angeles: University of California Press.

Lerdahl, Fred. 1988. "Cognitive Constraints on Compositional Systems." In *Cognitive Processes in Music*, ed. John Sloboda, 231–59. New York: Oxford University Press.

Lerdahl, Fred. 2001. *Tonal Pitch Space*. New York: Oxford University Press.

Lerdahl, Fred and Ray Jackendoff. 1983. *A Generative Theory of Tonal Music*. Cambridge, Mass.: MIT Press.

Lerner, Neil. 2004. "Review of *Copland Connotations*, ed. Peter Dickinson." *Music & Letters* 85(2): 332–35.

Lerner, Neil. 2009. "Music." In *Encyclopedia of American Disability History*, ed. Susan Burch, 638–39. New York: Facts on File.

Lerner, Neil and Joseph N. Straus. 2006. *Sounding Off: Theorizing Disability in Music*. New York: Routledge.

Lessem, Alan. 1997. "The Emigré Experience: Schoenberg in America." In *Constructive Dissonance: Arnold Schoenberg and the Transformations of Twentieth-Century Culture*, ed. Juliane Brand and Christopher Hailey, 58–70. Berkeley and Los Angeles: University of California Press.

Lewin, David. 1968. "Inversional Balance as an Organizing Force in Schoenberg's Music and Thought." *Perspectives of New Music* 6(2): 1–21.

Lewin, David. 1982–83. "Transformational Techniques in Atonal and Other Music Theories." *Perspectives of New Music* 21: 312–71.

Lewin, David. 1987. *Generalized Musical Intervals and Transformations*. New Haven, Conn.: Yale University Press.

Lewin, David. 1993. *Musical Form and Transformation: 4 Analytic Essays*. New Haven, Conn.: Yale University Press.

Lewin, David. 1997. "Some Notes on *Pierrot Lunaire*." In *Music Theory in Concept and Practice*, ed. James Baker, David Beach, and Jonathan Bernard, 433–58. Rochester, N.Y.: University of Rochester Press.

Lewis, Vicki. 1981. "Itzhak Perlman: Artist and Advocate." *Independent* 9(1): 8–11, 30–31

Lewis, Bradley. 2006. *Moving Beyond Prozac, DSM, and the New Psychiatry: The Birth of Postpsychiatry*. Ann Arbor: University of Michigan Press.

Linton, Simi. 1998. *Claiming Disability: Knowledge and Identity*. New York: New York University Press.

Linton, Simi. 2006. *My Body Politic: A Memoir*. Ann Arbor: University of Michigan Press.

Lockwood, Lewis. 1982. "'Eroica' Perspectives: Strategy and Design in the First Movement." In *Beethoven Studies*, vol. 3, ed. Alan Tyson, 85–96. Cambridge: Cambridge University Press.

Long, Marguerite. 1973. *At the Piano with Ravel*, ed. Pierre Laumonier, trans. Olive Senior-Ellis. London: Dent.

Longmore, Paul. 2003. *Why I Burned My Book and Other Essays on Disability*. Philadelphia: Temple University Press.

Longmore, Paul and Lauri Umansky. 2001. "Introduction: Disability History: From the Margins to the Mainstream." In *The New Disability History: American Perspectives*, ed. Paul Longmore and Lauri Umansky, 1–32. New York: New York University Press.

Lubet, Alex. 2004. "Tunes of Impairment: An Ethnomusicology of Disability." *Review of Disability Studies* 1(1): 133–56.

Macaskill, Mark. 2008. "Evelyn Glennie to Learn Sign Language at Age of 42." *London Times*, July 13, 2008.

MacMaster, Henry. 1928. *La folie de Robert Schumann*. Paris: Éditions N. Maloine.

Mairs, Nancy. 1996. *Waist-High in the World: A Life Among the Nondisabled*. Boston: Beacon Press.

Malone, Sean. 2000. "Glenn Gould's Imaginary Orchestra: Much Ado About Humming."Paper presented at the annual conference of the American Musicological Society and the Society for Music Theory, Toronto, 4 November 2000.

Maloney, Timothy. 2006. "Glenn Gould, Autistic Savant." In *Sounding Off: Theorizing Disability in Music*, ed. Neil Lerner and Joseph N. Straus, 121–36. New York: Routledge.

Marin, Oscar and David Perry. 1999. "Neurological Aspects of Music Perception and Performance." In *The Psychology of Music*, 2d ed, ed. Diana Deutsch, 653–724. San Diego, Calif.: Academic Press.

Marshall, Robert. 1976. "Bach the Progressive: Observations on His Later Works." *Musical Quarterly* 62(3): 313–57.

Marx, Adolf Bernhard. 1859. *Ludwig van Beethoven: Leben und Schaffen*, 2 vols. Berlin: Otto Janke; reprint, Hildesheim: Georg Olms, 1979.

Maus, Fred. 1993. "Masculine Discourse in Music Theory." *Perspectives of New Music* 31(2): 264–93.

Maus, Fred. 2010. "Somaesthetics of Music." *Action, Criticism, and Theory for Music Education* 9(1): 10–25.

McClary, Susan. 1993. "Music and Sexuality: On the Steblin/Solomon Debate." *Nineteenth-Century Music* 17/1: 83–88.

McFerran, Katrina, Ju-Young Lee, Megan Steele, and Andrea Bialocerkowski. 2009. "A Descriptive Review of the Literature (1990–2006) Addressing Music Therapy with People Who Have Disabilities." *Musica Humana* 1(1): 45–80.

McGeer, Victoria. 2004. "Autistic Self-Awareness." *Philosophy, Psychiatriy, and Psychology* 11(3): 235–51.

McLellan, Joseph. 1981. "Perlman to the Defense." *Washington Post*, March 19, 1981: D1, D14.

McRuer, Robert. 2002. "Compulsory Able-Bodiedness and Queer/Disabled Existence." In *Disability Studies: Enabling the Humanities*, ed. Sharon Snyder, Brenda Joe Brueggemann, and Rosemarie Garland-Thomson, 88–99. New York: Modern Language Association of America.

McRuer, Robert. 2006. *Crip Theory: Cultural Signs of Queerness and Disability.* New York: New York University Press.

Mead, Andrew. 1999. "Bodily Hearing: Physiological Metaphors and Musical Understanding." *Journal of Music Theory* 43(1): 1–19.

Micznik, Vera. 1996. "The Farewell Story of Mahler's Ninth Symphony." *Nineteenth-Century Music* 20(2): 144–66.

Miller, Leon K. 1987. "Sensitivity to Tonal Structure in a Developmentally Disabled Musical Savant." *Psychology of Music* 15: 76–89.

Miller, Leon K. 1989. *Musical Savants: Exceptional Skill in the Mentally Retarded.* Mahwah, N.J.: Lawrence Erlbaum Associates.

Mills, Bruce. 2008. "Autism and the Imagination." In *Autism and Representation*, ed. Mark Osteen, 117–32. New York: Routledge.

Mitchell, David and Sharon Snyder. 1997. "Introduction: Disability Studies and the Double Bind of Representation." In *The Body and Physical Difference: Discourses of Disability*, ed. David Mitchell and Sharon Snyder, 1–34. Ann Arbor: University of Michigan Press.

Mitchell, David and Sharon Snyder. 2000. *Narrative Prosthesis: Disability and the Dependencies of Discourse.* Ann Arbor: University of Michigan Press.

Morgan, Robert. 1992. *Anthology of Twentieth-Century Music.* New York: Norton.

Morris, Rebecca. 2009. "Universal Design and Adaptive Equipment: Ideas and Solutions for Music Schools." *Music Theory Online* 15(3).

Morris, Robert. 1995. "Compositional Spaces and Other Territories." *Perspectives of New Music* 33(1–2): 328–58.

Moss, Stephen. 2000. "'I'm lucky. Everyone can see my disability': Thomas Quasthoff was born a 'Thalidomide baby': But he has a voice sublime enough to overcome any prejudice." *Guardian*, October 20, 2000.

Mostel, Raphael. 2005. "A Demanding Composer Meets his Orchestral Match." *Jewish Daily Forward* (online edition of the *Forward*), November 25, 2005.

Mottron, Laurent, Isabelle Peretz, Sylvie Belleville, and Sophie Blanchet. 1999. "*Absolute Pitch in Autism: A Case-Study.*" *Neurocase* 5: 485–501.

Murray, Stuart. 2008. *Representing Autism: Culture, Narrative, Fascination.* Liverpool, England: Liverpool University Press.

Nabokov, Nicholas. 1951. *Old Friends and New Music.* London: Hamish Hamilton.

Nazeer, Kamran. 2006. *Send in the Idiots: Stories from the Other Side of Autism.* New York: Bloomsbury.

Neff, Severine. 2001. "Reinventing the Organic Artwork: Schoenberg's Changing Image of Tonal Form." In *Schoenberg and Words: The Modernist Years*, ed. Charlotte Cross and Russell Berman, 287–307. New York: Garland.

Neumayr, Anton. 1994. *Music and Medicine, vol. 1 (Haydn, Mozart, Beethoven, Schubert): Notes on Their Lives, Works, and Medical Histories*, trans. Bruce Cooper Clarke. Bloomington, Ill.: Medi-Ed Press.

Neumayr, Anton. 1995. *Music and Medicine, vol. 2 (Hummel, Weber, Mendelssohn, Schumann, Brahms, Bruckner): Notes on Their Lives, Works, and Medical Histories*, trans. Bruce Cooper Clarke. Bloomington, Ill.: Medi-Ed Press.

Neumayr, Anton. 1997. *Music and Medicine, vol. 3 (Chopin, Smetana, Tchaikovsky, Mahler): Notes on Their Lives, Works, and Medical Histories*, trans. David J. Parent. Bloomington, Ill.: Medi-Ed Press.

Neumeyer, David. 2006. "Description and Interpretation: Fred Lerdahl's *Tonal Pitch Space* and Linear Analysis." *Music Analysis* 25(1–2): 201–30.

Newman, William. 1983. *The Sonata Since Beethoven*, 3d ed. New York: Norton.

Nichols, Robert. 1976. "Delius as I Knew Him." In *A Delius Companion*, ed. Christopher Redwood, 113–116. London: John Calder.

Niecks, Frederick. 1925. *Robert Schumann*. London: Dent.

Nochlin, Linda. 1994. *The Body in Pieces: The Fragment as a Metaphor of Modernity*. New York: Thames & Hudson.

Nordau, Max. 1892/1993. *Degeneration*, trans. George L. Mosse. Lincoln: University of Nebraska Press.

Norden, Martin. 1996. *The Cinema of Isolation: A History of Physical Disability in the Movies*. New Brunswick, N.J.: Rutgers University Press.

Notley, Margaret. 2007. *Lateness and Brahms: Music and Culture in the Twilight of Viennese Liberalism*. New York: Oxford University Press.

Nupen, Christopher, dir. 2007. "Itzhak Perlman: Virtuoso Violinist (I Know I Played Every Note)." Allegro Films.

O'Connell, Deirdre. 2009. *The Ballad of Blind Tom*. New York: Overlook Press.

O'Brien, Ruth. 2005. *Bodies in Revolt: Gender, Disability, and a Workplace Ethic of Care*. New York: Routledge.

Ockelford, Adam. 2007. *In the Key of Genius: The Extraordinary Life of Derek Paravicini*. London: Hutchinson.

Orenstein, Arbie, ed. 1990. *A Ravel Reader: Correspondence, Articles, Interviews*. New York: Columbia University Press.

O'Shea, John. 1990. *Was Mozart Poisoned? Medical Investigations into the Lives of the Great Composers*. New York: St. Martin's Press.

Oster, Andrew. 2006. "Melisma as Malady: Cavalli's *Il Giasone* (1649) and Opera's Earliest Stuttering Role." In *Sounding Off: Theorizing Disability in Music*, ed. Neil Lerner and Joseph N. Straus, 157–72. New York: Routledge.

Ostwald, Peter. 1985. *Schumann: The Inner Voices of a Musical Genius*. Boston: Northeastern University Press.

Ostwald, Peter. 1997. *Glenn Gould: The Ecstasy and Tragedy of Genius*. New York: Norton.

Oteri, Frank. 2008. "Gabriela Lena Frank: Composite Identity (Hearing Things Differently)." NewMusicBox.org, accessed October 19, 2010. http://www.newmusicbox.org/article.nmbx?id=5517

Oulibicheff, Alexandre. 1857. *Beethoven, Ses critiques et ses glossateurs*. Leipzig, Germany: F. A. Brockhaus.

Oyler, Philip T. 1972. "Delius at Grèz." *The Musical Times* 113(1551): 444–47.

Padden, Carol and Tom Humphries. 1988. *Deaf in America: Voices from a Culture*. Cambridge, Mass.: Harvard University Press.

Payne, Anthony. 1961–1962. "Delius's Stylistic Development." *Tempo* 60: 6–25.

Peles, Steven. 2004. "'Ist Alles Eins': Schoenberg and Symmetry." *Music Theory Spectrum* 26(1): 57–86.

Perle, George. 1991. *Serial Composition and Atonality*, 6th ed. Berkeley and Los Angeles: University of California Press.

Perle, George. 1996. *Twelve-Tone Tonality*, 2d ed. Berkeley and Los Angeles: University of California Press.

Pezzl, Johann. 1923. *Skizze von Wien; ein Kultur und Sittenbild aus der josefinischen Zeit. Mit Einleitung, Anmerkungen und Register*, ed. Gustav Gugitz and Anton Schlossar. Graz, Austria: Leykam.

Phillips, Gordon. 2004. *The Blind in British Society: Charity, State and Community, c. 1780–1930*. Aldershot, England: Ashgate.

Pick, Daniel. 1989. *Faces of Degeneration: A European Disorder, c. 1848-c. 1918*. Cambridge: Cambridge University Press.

Pollack, Howard. 1999. *Aaron Copland: The Life and Work of an Uncommon Man*. New York: Henry Holt.

Poore, Carol. 2009. *Disability in Twentieth-Century German Culture*. Ann Arbor: University of Michigan Press.

Porter, Roy. 2002. *Madness: A Brief History*. Oxford: Oxford University Press.

Powell, Nicholas. 1974. *The Sacred Spring: The Arts in Vienna, 1898–1918*. New York: Graphic Society.

Pring, Linda et al. 2008. "Melody and Pitch Processing in Five Musical Savants with Congenital Blindness." *Perception* 37(2): 290–307.

Prout, Ebenezer. 1895. *Applied Forms: a Sequel to "Musical Form."* London: Augener.

Quaglia, Bruce. 2007. "Beethoven's *Pathétique* Sonata, First Movement, and the Normal Body: The Idea of Formal Prosthesis." Paper presented to the Rocky Mountain Chapter of the American Musicological Society.

Quasthoff, Thomas. 2008. *The Voice: A Memoir*, trans. Kirsten Stoldt Wittenborn. New York: Pantheon.

Quinn, Ian. 2006. "Minimal Challenges: Process Music and the Uses of Formalist Analysis," *Contemporary Music Review* 25(3): 283–94.

Radden, Jennifer, ed. 2002. *The Nature of Melancholy: From Aristotle to Kristeva*. New York: Oxford University Press.

Ratner, Leonard. 1980. *Classic Music: Expression, Form and Style*. New York: Schirmer Books.

Reisler, Jim. 2002. *Voices of the Oral Deaf: Fourteen Role Models Speak Out*. Jefferson, N.C.: McFarland.

Riedelsheimer, Thomas, dir. 2004. *Touch the Sound: A Sound Journey with Evelyn Glennie*. New Video Group.

Riis, Thomas. 1976. "The Cultivated White Tradition and Black Music in Nineteenth-Century America: A Discussion of Some Articles in J. S. Dwight's Journal of Music." *The Black Perspective in Music* 4/2: 156–76.

Révész, Geza. 1925. *The Psychology of a Musical Prodigy*. New York: Harcourt & Brace.

Rodas, Julia Miele. 2008. "'On the Spectrum': Rereading Contact and Affect in *Jane Eyre*." *Nineteenth-Century Gender Studies* 4(2).

Rolland, Romain. 1956. *Beethoven the Creator*, trans. Ernest Newman. Reprint, New York: Dover, 1929.

Rosen, Charles. 1972. *The Classical Style: Haydn, Mozart, Beethoven*. New York: Norton.

Rosen, Charles. 1975. *Arnold Schoenberg*. New York: Viking.

Rosen, Charles. 1988. *Sonata Forms*, revised ed. New York: Norton.

Rosen, Charles. 1995. *The Romantic Generation*. Cambridge, Mass.: Harvard University Press.

Rothstein, William. 1989. *Phrase Rhythm in Tonal Music.* New York: Schirmer Books.

Rothstein, William. 1990. "Rhythmic Displacement and Rhythmic Normalization." In *Trends in Schenkerian Analysis,* ed. Allen Cadwallader, 87–113. New York: Schirmer Books.

Rothstein, Mervyn. 1993. "For the Disabled, Some Progress." *New York Times,* October 24, 1993: R1, R11.

Rowden, Terry. 2009. *The Songs of Blind Folk: African-American Musicians and the Cultures of Blindness.* Ann Arbor: University of Michigan Press.

Rubsamen, Walter. 1951. "Schoenberg in America." *Musical Quarterly* 37(4): 469–89.

Sacks, Oliver. 1995. *An Anthropologist on Mars: Seven Paradoxical Tales.* New York: Alfred A. Knopf.

Sacks, Oliver. 2007. *Musicophilia: Tales of Music and the Brain.* New York: Alfred A. Knopf.

Said, Edward. 2006. *On Late Style: Music and Literature Against the Grain.* New York: Pantheon Books.

Sams, Eric. 1971. "Schumann's Hand Injury." *Musical Times* 112: 1156–59.

Sams, Eric. 1980. "Schubert's Illness Re-examined." *Musical Times* 121: 15–22.

Sandahl, Carrie. 2003. "Queering the Crip or Cripping the Queer: Intersections of Queer and Crip Identities in Solo Autobiographical Performance." *GLQ: A Journal of Gay and Lesbian Studies* 9: 25–56.

Sandahl, Carrie and Philip Auslander, ed. 2005. *Bodies in Commotion: Disability and Performance.* Ann Arbor: University of Michigan Press.

Saslaw, Janna. 1996. "Forces, Containers, and Paths: The Role of Body-Derived Image Schemas in the Conceptualization of Music." *Journal of Music Theory* 40(2): 217–44.

Saslaw, Janna. 1997–98. "Life Forces: Conceptual Structures in Schenker's *Free Composition* and Schoenberg's *The Musical Idea*." *Theory and Practice* 22–23: 17–34.

Schenker, Heinrich. 1935. *Free Composition (Der freie Satz),* trans. and ed. Ernst Oster. New York: Longman, 1979.

Schenker, Heinrich. 1910–22. *Counterpoint,* ed. John Rothgeb, trans. John Rothgeb and Jurgen Thym. New York: Schirmer Books, 1987.

Schenker, Heinrich. 1996. "Further Consideration of the Urlinie: II." In *The Masterwork in Music,* vol. 2, ed. William Drabkin, trans. John Rothgeb, 1–19. Cambridge: Cambridge University Press.

Schenker, Heinrich. 1997. "Rameau or Beethoven? Creeping Paralysis or Spiritual Potency in Music?" In *The Masterwork in Music,* vol. 3, ed. William Drabkin, trans. Ian Bent, 1–9. Cambridge: Cambridge University Press.

Schering, Arnold. 1933. "Die *Eroica,* eine Homer-Symphonie Beethovens?" *Neues Beethoven Jahrbuch* 5: 159–77.

Scherzinger, Martin. 1997. "Anton Webern and the Concept of Symmetrical Inversion: A Reconsideration on the Terrain of Gender." *repercussions* 6(2): 63–147.

Schleuning, Peter. 1987. "Beethoven in alter Deutung: Der 'neue Weg' mit der 'Sinfonia eroica.'" *Archiv für Musikwissenschaft* 44: 165–94.

Schoenberg, Arnold. 1967. *Fundamentals of Musical Composition,* ed. Gerald Strang and Leonard Stein. London: Faber & Faber.

Schoenberg, Arnold. 1911. *Theory of Harmony,* trans. Roy Carter. Berkeley and Los Angeles: University of California Press, 1978.

Schoenberg, Arnold. 1912. "The Relationship to the Text." In *Style and Idea: Selected Writings of Arnold Schoenberg,* ed. Leonard Stein, trans. Leo Black, 141–45. Berkeley and Los Angeles: University of California Press, 1984.

Schoenberg, Arnold. 1941. "Composition with Twelve Tones." In *Style and Idea: Selected Writings of Arnold Schoenberg,* ed. Leonard Stein, trans. Leo Black, 214–44. Berkeley and Los Angeles: University of California Press, 1984.

Schoenberg, Arnold. 1946. "New Music, Outmoded Music." In *Style and Idea: Selected Writings of Arnold Schoenberg*, ed. Leonard Stein, trans. Leo Black, 113–23. London: Faber & Faber, 1984.

Schoenberg, Arnold. 1948. "Gustav Mahler." In *Style and Idea: Selected Writings of Arnold Schoenberg*, ed. Leonard Stein, trans. Leo Black, 449–72. Berkeley and Los Angeles: University of California Press, 1984.

Schoenberg, Arnold. 1995. *The Musical Idea and the Logic, Technique, and Art of Its Presentation*, ed. and trans. Patricia Carpenter and Severine Neff. New York: Columbia University Press.

Schorske, Carl. 1981. *Fin-de-Siècle Vienna: Politics and Culture*. New York: Random House.

Schreibman, Laura. 2005. *The Science and Fiction of Autism*. Cambridge, Mass.: Harvard University Press.

Schwarz, K. Robert. 1999. "A Composer Freed by Opera to be Tonal and Tuneful." *New York Times* May 2, 1999.

Scully, Jackie Leach. 2008. *Disability Bioethics: Moral Bodies, Moral Difference*. Lanham, Md.: Rowman & Littlefield.

Serafine, Mary Louise. 1988. *Music as Cognition: The Development of Thought in Sound*. New York: Columbia University Press.

Shakespeare, Tom. 2006. *Disability Rights and Wrongs*. London: Routledge.

Sheinberg, Esti. 2000. *Irony, Satire, Parody and the Grotesque in the Music of Shostakovich: A Theory of Musical Incongruities*. Aldershot, England: Ashgate.

Siebers, Tobin. 2008. *Disability Theory*. Ann Arbor: University of Michigan Press.

Siebers, Tobin. 2010. *Disability Aesthetics*. Ann Arbor: University of Michigan Press.

Silvers, Anita and Leslie Francis. 2010. "Thinking About the Good: Reconfiguring Liberal Metaphysics (or Not) for People with Cognitive Disabilities." In *Cognitive Disability and its Challenge to Moral Philosophy*, ed. Eva Kittay and Licia Carlson, 237–60. Oxford: Wiley-Blackwell.

Singer, Julie. 2010. "Playing by Ear: Compensation, Reclamation, and Prosthesis in Fourteenth-Century Song." In *Disability in the Middle Ages: Reconsiderations and Reverberations*, ed. Joshua R. Eyler, 39–52. Aldershot, England: Ashgate.

Sipe, Thomas. 1992. *Interpreting Beethoven: History, Aesthetics, and Critical Reception*. Ph. D. diss., University of Pennsylvania, Philadelphia.

Sipe, Thomas. 1998. *Beethoven: Eroica Symphony*. Cambridge: Cambridge University Press.

Sloboda, John. 2005. *Exploring the Musical Mind: Cognition, Emotion, Ability, Function*. Oxford: Oxford University Press.

Sly, Gordon. 2001. "Schubert's Innovations in Sonata Form: Compositional Logic and Structural Interpretation." *Journal of Music Theory* 45(1): 119–43.

Smith, Bonnie G. and Beth Hutchison, eds. 2004. *Gendering Disability*. New Brunswick, N.J.: Rutgers University Press.

Smith, Peter H. 2006. "Harmonic Cross-Reference and the Dialectic of Articulation and Continuity in Sonata Expositions of Schubert and Brahms." *Journal of Music Theory* 50(2): 143–80.

Solomon, Maynard. 1989. "Franz Schubert and the Peacocks of Benvenuto Cellini." *Nineteenth-Century Music* 12: 193–206.

Solomon, Maynard. 1998. *Beethoven*, 2d ed. New York: Schirmer Books.

Solomon, Maynard. 2003. *Late Beethoven: Music, Thought, Imagination*. Berkeley and Los Angeles: University of California Press.

Sonenberg, Daniel. 2003. *"Who in the World She Might Be": A Contextual and Stylistic Approach to the Early Music of Joni Mitchell*. Ph.D. diss., City University of New York, New York.

Sontag, Susan. 1978. *Illness as Metaphor*. New York: Farrar, Straus & Giroux.

Southall, Geneva Handy. 1979. *Blind Tom: The Post Civil-war Enslavement of a Black Musical Genius*. Minneapolis, Minn.: Challenge Books.

Southall, Geneva Handy. 1983. *The Continuing Enslavement of Blind Tom, the Black Pianist-Composer (1865–1887)*. Minneapolis, Minn.: Challenge Books.

Southall, Geneva Handy. 1999. *Blind Tom, The Black Pianist Composer: Continually Enslaved*. Lanham, Md.: Scarecrow Press.

Stein, Erwin, ed. 1965. *Arnold Schoenberg Letters*, trans. Eithne Wilkins and Ernst Kaiser. New York: St. Martin's Press.

Stevens, Denis. 1961. "Master Francis of Florence." *Musical Times* 102(1416): 90–91.

Stevens, Halsey. 1993. *The Life and Music of Béla Bartók*, 3d ed. Oxford: Clarendon Press.

Stiker, Henri-Jacques. 2000. *A History of Disability*, trans. William Sayers. Ann Arbor: University of Michigan Press.

Stoecker, Philip. 2003. *Studies in Post-tonal Symmetry: A Transformational Approach*. Ph.D. diss., City University of New York, New York.

Stone, Anne. 2009. "The Story in the Song: Autobiography and Lyric in the works of 'Franciscus cecus de Florentia' (a.k.a. Francesco Landini)." Unpublished paper.

Stras, Laurie. 2006. "The Organ of the Soul: Voice, Damage, and Affect." In *Sounding Off: Theorizing Disability in Music*, ed. Neil Lerner and Joseph N. Straus, 173–84. New York: Routledge.

Stras, Laurie. 2009. "Sing a Song of Difference: Connie Boswell and a Discourse of Disability in Jazz." *Popular Music* 28(3): 297–322.

Straus, Joseph N. 1990. *Remaking the Past: Musical Modernism and the Influence of the Tonal Tradition*. Cambridge, Mass.: Harvard University Press.

Straus, Joseph N. 2001. *Stravinsky's Late Music*. Cambridge: Cambridge University Press.

Straus, Joseph N. 2006a. "Normalizing the Abnormal: Disability in Music and Music Theory." *Journal of the American Musicological Society* 59(1): 113–84.

Straus, Joseph N. 2006b. "Inversional Balance and the 'Normal' Body in the Music of Arnold Schoenberg and Anton Webern." In *Sounding Off: Theorizing Disability in Music*, ed. Neil Lerner and Joseph N. Straus, 257–68. New York: Routledge.

Straus, Joseph N. 2008. "Disability and Late Style in Music." *Journal of Musicology* 25(1): 3–45.

Straus, Joseph N. 2010. "Autism as Culture." In *The Disability Studies Reader*, 3d ed., ed. Lennard Davis, 535–62. New York: Routledge.

Stravinsky, Igor and Robert Craft. 1966. *Themes and Episodes*. New York: Alfred A. Knopf.

Stravinsky, Vera and Robert Craft. 1978. *Stravinsky in Pictures and Documents*. New York: Simon & Schuster.

Sullivan, J. W. N. 1927. *Beethoven: His Spiritual Development*. New York: Alfred A. Knopf.

Tallián, Tibor. 1995. "Bartók's Reception in America, 1940–1945," trans. Peter Laki. In *Bartók and His World*, ed. Peter Laki, 101–18. Princeton, N.J.: Princeton University Press.

Taruskin, Richard. 1996. *Stravinsky and the Russian Traditions*. Berkeley and Los Angeles: University of California Press.

Taruskin, Richard. 2005. *The Oxford History of Western Music*. Vol. 1. *The Earliest Notations to the Sixteenth Century*. Vol. 2. *Music in the Seventeenth and Eighteenth Centuries*. Vol. 3. *Music in the Nineteenth Century*. New York: Oxford University Press.

Taylor, Ronald. 1982. *Robert Schumann: His Life and Work*. New York: Universe.

Temperley, David. 2007. *Music and Probability*. Cambridge, Mass.: MIT Press.

Thomas, Carol and Mairian Corker. 2002. "A Journey Around the Social Model." In *Disability/Postmodernity: Embodying Disability Theory*, ed. Mairian Corker and Tom Shakespeare, 18–31. London: Continuum.

Tick, Judith. 2000. "The Music of Aaron Copland." In *Aaron Copland's America: A Cultural Perspective*, ed. Gail Levin and Judith Tick, 128–64. New York: Watson-Guptill.

Tolstoy, Leo. 1869/2007. *War and Peace*. Trans. Richard Pevear and Larissa Volokhonsky. New York: Alfred A. Knopf.

Tommasini, Anthony. 2004. "It's the Vocal Chords that Matter Most." *New York Times*, January 28, 2004: E1, E6.

Tovey, Donald Francis. 1935. *Essays in Musical Analysis: Symphonies*. London: Oxford University Press.

Tovey, Donald Francis. 1949a. "Some Aspects of Beethoven's Art Forms." In *The Main Stream of Music and Other Essays*, 271–97. New York: Oxford University Press.

Tovey, Donald Francis. 1949b. "Normality and Freedom in Music." In *The Main Stream of Music and Other Essays*, 183–95. New York: Oxford University Press.

Treffert, D. A. 1988. "The idiot savant: A review of the syndrome." *American Journal of Psychiatry* 145: 563–72.

Tunbridge, Laura. 2007. *Schumann's Late Style*. Cambridge: Cambridge University Press.

Updike, John. 2006. "Late Works." *The New Yorker*, August 7, 2006.

Van den Toorn, Pieter. 1983. *The Music of Igor Stravinsky*. New Haven, Conn.: Yale University Press.

Veditz, George. 1912. "President's Message." In *Proceedings of the Ninth Convention of the National Association of the Deaf and the Third World's Congress of the Deaf, 1910*. Philadelphia: Philocophus Press.

Vogel, Carol. 2009. "Adapting a House for Itzhak Perlman." *New York Times*, January 30, 2009.

Walker, Alan. 1976. *Schumann*. London: Faber & Faber.

Wallace, Robin. 1986. *Beethoven's Critics: Aesthetic Dilemmas and Resolutions during the Composer's Lifetime*. Cambridge: Cambridge University Press.

Walsh, Stephen. 2006. *Stravinsky, The Second Exile: France and America, 1934–1971*. New York: Alfred A. Knopf.

Ward, W. Dixon. 1999. "Absolute Pitch." In *The Psychology of Music*, 2d ed., ed. Diana Deutsch, 265–98. San Diego, Calif.: Academic Press.

Watters, Ethan. 2010. "The Americanization of Mental Illness." *New York Times Magazine*. January 10, 2010, 38–45.

Webster, James. 1978–79. "Schubert's Sonata Forms and Brahms's First Maturity." *Nineteenth-Century Music* 2: 18–35 and 3: 52–71.

Webster, James. 2001. "Sonata Form." In *The New Grove Dictionary of Music and Musicians*, 2d ed., edited by Stanley Sadie, 23, 687–701. London: Macmillan.

Wendell, Susan. 1996. *The Rejected Body: Feminist Philosophical Reflections on the Disabled Body*. New York: Routledge.

Wendell, Susan. 1997. "Toward a Feminist Theory of Disability." In *The Disability Studies Reader*, ed, Lennard Davis, 260–78. New York: Routledge.

Westergaard, Peter. 1996. "Geometries of Sounds in Time," *Music Theory Spectrum* 18(1): 1–21.

Whalen, Robert Weldon. 1984. *Bitter Wounds: German Victims of the Great War, 1914–1939*. Ithaca, N.Y.: Cornell University Press.

White, Patrick. 2003. "Sex Education; Or, How The Blind Became Heterosexual." *GLQ: A Journal of Lesbian and Gay Studies* 9(1–2): 133–47.

Whittall, Arnold. 2001. "Schoenberg Since 1951: Overlapping Opposites." *Musical Times* 142(1876): 11–20.

Wiegman, Robyn, ed. 1995. *American Anatomies: Theorizing Race and Gender*. Durham, N.C.: Duke University Press.

Wills, David. 1995. *Prosthesis*. Stanford, Calif.: Stanford University Press.

Winzer, Margaret. 1997. "Disability and Society Before the Eighteenth Century: Dread and Despair." In *The Disability Studies Reader*, ed. Lennard Davis, 75–109. London: Routledge.

Woo, Judy. 2010. *Focal Dystonia in Pianists*. Ph.D. diss., City University of New York, New York.

Wood, Elizabeth. 2009. "On Deafness and Musical Creativity: The Case of Ethel Smyth." *Musical Quarterly* 92(1–2): 33–69.

Wood, Leonard, ed. 1939. *The Works of Francesco Landini*. Cambridge, Mass.: Medieval Academy of America.

Zbikowski, Lawrence. 1997–98. "*Des Herzraums Abschied*: Mark Johnson's Theory of Embodied Knowledge and Music Theory." *Theory and Practice* 22–23: 1–16.

Zbikowski, Lawrence. 2002. *Conceptualizing Music: Cognitive Structure, Theory, and Analysis*. New York: Oxford University Press.

Zbikowski, Lawrence. 2009. "Musicology, Cognitive Science, and Metaphor: Reflections on Michael Spitzer's *Metaphor and Musical Thought*." *Musica Humana* 1(1): 81–104.

INDEX

Verdi, Giuseppe, 6, 142
Vocal disfluency, 126

Wagner, Richard, 28, 142
Webern, Anton, 73–81, 86, 122, 123
Webern, Anton, works of:
    Bagatelle, op. 9, No. 5, 74, 76
    Orchestra Pieces, op. 10, 123
    String Quartet, op. 5, no. 2, 74, 76,
      122 n. 36

Wiggins, Thomas (Thomas Bethune; Tom
    Wiggins; "Blind Tom"), 132–137,
    140, 148, 165
Wilde, Oscar, 77
Wittgenstein, Paul, 126
Wonder, Stevie, 131
World Health Organization (WHO),
    3 n. 1

Zemlinsky, Alexander von, 77, 104 n. 1

Made in the USA
San Bernardino, CA
02 April 2015